BEHAVIORAL ADDICTION

Screening, Assessment, and Treatment

An-Pyng Sun

Larry Ashley

Lesley Dickson

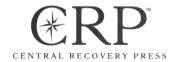

CENTRAL RECOVERY PRESS

Central Recovery Press (CRP) is committed to publishing exceptional materials addressing addiction treatment, recovery, and behavioral healthcare topics, including original and quality books, audio/visual communications, and web-based new media. Through a diverse selection of titles, we seek to contribute a broad range of unique resources for professionals, recovering individuals and their families, and the general public.

For more information, visit www.centralrecoverypress.com.

Central Recovery Press, Las Vegas, NV 89129

Publisher: Central Recovery Press
           3321 N. Buffalo Drive
           Las Vegas, NV 89129

18 17 16 15 14 13   1 2 3 4 5

ISBN-13: 978-1-936290-97-0 (paper)
ISBN-13: 978-1-937612-05-4 (e-book)

Chapter Three adapted from "Pathological Gambling: A General Overview," by Larry L. Ashley and Karmen Boehlke, *Journal of Psychoactive Drugs* Volume 44, Issue 1, pp 27–37. Reprinted with permission of Taylor and Francis (http://www.tandfonline.com).

Publisher's Note: This book contains general information about various manifestations of addiction, assessment tools, and suggested treatments. The information is not medical advice and should not be treated as such. Central Recovery Press makes no representations or warranties in relation to the medical information in this book; this book is not an alternative to medical advice from your doctor or other professional healthcare provider. If you have any specific questions about any medical matter you should consult your doctor or other professional healthcare provider. If you think you or someone close to you may be suffering from any medical condition, you should seek immediate medical attention. You should never delay seeking medical advice, disregard medical advice, or discontinue medical treatment because of information in this or any book.

Cover design and interior design and layout by
Tom Carling, Carling Design, Inc.

Contents

CHAPTER ONE
Historical Background and the Trend Today   9

CHAPTER TWO
The Brain and Addiction   35

CHAPTER THREE
Gambling Addiction   45

CHAPTER FOUR
Sexual Addiction   75

CHAPTER FIVE
Eating Disorders   99

CHAPTER SIX
Impulse Control Disorders   115

CHAPTER SEVEN
Internet Addiction   131

Appendix   163

Chapter Notes   185

Glossary   221

To help you better understand some of the terminology in this book,
a glossary has been added for your reference. Words that are included
in the glossary are italicized in the text.

Bibliography   227

1

Historical Background of Behavioral Addiction and the Trend Today

An-Pyng Sun, PhD, LCSW

Historically, behavioral addiction and its treatment have been neglected by both the general public and mental health professionals, who have focused on substance addiction problems. Such a trend may be forced to change, no matter how slowly, because of enormous social and environmental changes, as well as the strides made in the fields of scientific research in the past several decades. These social and environmental changes have facilitated and heightened certain behavioral addiction problems. For example, there was exponential growth in the number of fast-food restaurants in the United States from about 600 in 1958 to 140,000 by 1980, and to an estimated 222,000 in 2010.[1] One of the factors contributing to the corresponding obesity epidemic may be binge eating/food addiction as the restaurants provide easy and affordable access to high consumption of palatable foods.[2, 3] In addition, the wide availability of Internet access in the past couple of decades has dramatically affected many people's lives. The "digital dope" epidemics in many countries, especially prevalent in

9

some Asian countries, not only relate to a new "Internet use disorder," but also new forms of old addictions, including Internet pornography addiction and online gambling addiction.

At the same time, the advance in scientific research has allowed us to better understand behavioral addiction, as well as its commonalities to and close relationship with substance addiction. For example, advanced technologies, such as functional magnetic resonance imaging, enable scientists and researchers to map the human brain and the functions of its various regions and observe the process of how our brain determines our behavior,[4] which leads to advanced knowledge regarding both substance and behavioral addictions.

Frequently, people may talk about how vicious substance abuse and dependence are and that a person may die from an overdose of heroin or alcohol; seldom do people talk about how an "overdose" of food consumption or Internet use could be lethal (other than sporadic cases reported by the media). Likewise, a teenager would tell us that students will be suspended from school if they use alcohol and/or other drugs (AOD), whereas nobody will be kicked out of school because of their excessive use of the Internet, engaging in dieting or binge eating, or their overspending habit. Similarly, although substance use disorders and nonsubstance behavioral addictions are both considered to be related to impulse-control problems in the *Diagnostic Statistical Manual (DSM) IV*, they have been grouped under different classifications— one in the category of "Substance-Related Disorders" (SRD) and the other in the category of "Impulse-Control Disorders Not Elsewhere Classified" (ICDNEC). The SRD chapter in the *DSM-IV-TR* is 105 pages, whereas the ICDNEC chapter is only fifteen pages.[5] Although there may be multiple reasons for the discrepancy, it shows the tendency of a de-emphasis on behavioral addiction. Furthermore, we have far fewer treatment programs specifically designed for clients with behavioral addiction than for clients with substance addiction.

Federal funding sources usually encourage substance addiction research, whereas seldom do they call for or sponsor applications for behavioral addiction research. The addiction treatment curricula offered in many universities accentuate substance addiction content rather than behavioral addiction. Without a doubt, behavioral addiction has been underidentified, undertreated, and understudied.

Society's greater emphasis on substance addiction than on behavioral addiction may be partly attributable to the perceived lower prevalence of behavioral addiction than of substance addiction. Another factor could be the belief that many abused drugs are illegal and therefore vicious and harmful, and that excessive drinking may pose hazards to public health such as drunk driving. On the other hand, society may view many behavioral addictions—such as food addiction (binge-eating disorders), hypersexual disorder, Internet use disorder, pathological gambling, or compulsive shopping— as extensions of normal human needs and behavior, and are therefore personal lifestyles or less harmful leisure activities. Not only is behavioral addiction minimized by the general public, but also some mental health professionals and scholars fear that the identification and targeting of behavioral addiction may pathologize everyday life behavior and create "diagnostic inflation" and "false epidemics."[6]

Before discussing why it is important to call attention to nonsubstance behavioral addiction and its treatment, it is helpful to first clarify the concepts of addiction, impulse-control disorder, and obsessive-compulsive disorder; introduce the historical background and context of addiction and impulse-control disorders in the *DSM-IV* and other literature; and present the recent new trend with respect to bringing substance addiction and nonsubstance behavioral addiction together under one umbrella, including the changes proposed by the various *DSM-5* work groups, as well as the controversy over whether and how different types of addictions and addiction-related disorders should be reconceptualized and reclassified.

Addiction vs. Impulse-Control Disorder vs. Obsessive-Compulsive Disorder

According to the American Society of Addiction Medicine (ASAM), addiction is a chronic disease that involves maladaptation and dysfunction of brain circuitries responsible for reward, memory, and motivation.[7] ASAM suggests that people with addiction problems may pathologically pursue relief and/or reward by means of substance use and other behavioral engagement and manifest negative implications biologically, psychologically, socially, and spiritually.[8] ASAM's definition of addiction appears to be consistent with the definition held by the National Institute on Drug Abuse (NIDA).[9] Based on a systematic literature review, Sussman and Sussman suggest that addiction includes five elements: "engagement in the behavior to achieve appetitive effects," "preoccupation with the behavior," "temporary satiation," "loss of control," and "suffering negative consequences."[10]

For impulse-control disorder (ICD), *DSM-IV-TR* suggests its essential feature to be an individual's inability to resist a drive, temptation, or impulse to carry out an act that is detrimental to the individual or to others.[11] The *DSM-IV-TR* additionally stated that most disorders listed in its section of Impulse-Control Disorder Not Elsewhere Classified possess the characteristics that the individual experiences an increasing sense of arousal or tension before executing the act and feels relief, gratification, or pleasure when executing the act.[12]

On the other hand, the *DSM-IV-TR* defined obsessive-compulsive disorder (OCD) as a person's repetitive and persistent attempts to use behaviors or mental acts to neutralize his or her persistent obsessions that are experienced as inappropriate and intrusive and that cause significant distress or anxiety in the person.[13] The *DSM-IV-TR* further explained that although some behaviors and activities—such as substance use, gambling, eating, and sexual behavior—tend to be referred to as being "compulsive" when being performed excessively, they should not be considered to be "compulsions" in the *DSM* because they usually provide pleasure and the person would oppose it only in the case of later subsequent adverse consequences.[14]

From the above three definitions, perhaps we can infer that a) in general, behavioral addiction can be conceptualized similarly with ICD because they both are ego-syntonic, or pleasure-seeking, in nature; b) not all ICDs are addictions because some of them may or may not involve focusing on pleasure-seeking, for example, intermittent explosive disorder does not share core characteristics with substance addiction[15] and individuals afflicted with hair-pulling disorder (trichotillomania) do not necessarily experience an urge before pulling and gratification during or after pulling;[16] c) in general, both behavioral addiction and ICD should be classified separately from OCD because the two former are ego-syntonic in nature whereas OCD is ego-dystonic, which focuses on harm avoidance and is opposite to ego-syntonic; and d) some ICDs may be closer to the family of OCD, that is, Obsessive-Compulsive Spectrum Disorder, or other categories of disorders than the category of addiction.

Fontenelle and colleagues said that many laymen use the expressions of ICD, OCD, and addictive behaviors interchangeably and that scientists and clinicians have attempted to disentangle the underlying concepts of these three entities, but the relationships among them are not that straightforward. They may overlap with respect to phenomenology, family history, comorbidity, neurochemistry, neurocognition, and neurocircuitry.[17] Although many researchers suggest independent categorizations between ICD and OCD in general, they emphasize that more research is needed as our understanding of the relationships between addiction, ICD, and OCD so far may have been compromised because of the limited research on ICD and OCD.[18]

The Historical Background of Addiction and the *DSM-IV*

The *DSM-IV* does not use the term "addiction"; substance addiction is close to its classification of Substance-Related Disorders (SRD), which includes substance use disorders (substance dependence and substance abuse) and substance-induced disorders (e.g., substance intoxication, substance withdrawal, and substance-induced mental disorders that are included elsewhere in the manual). Nonsubstance behavioral addiction is close to its classification of Impulse-Control Disorders Not Elsewhere Classified (ICDNEC), which includes Pathological Gambling, Intermittent Explosive Disorder, Kleptomania, Pyromania, Trichotillomania, and Impulse-Control Disorder Not Otherwise Specified (ICDNOS). Its category of ICDNOS may further include Internet use disorder, compulsive sexual or hypersexual disorder (nonparaphilic hypersexuality), compulsive-impulsive buying, compulsive-impulsive eating, and compulsive-impulsive skin-picking.

Disorders of animal/inanimate hoarding, impulsive-compulsive exercising, compulsive tanning, and workaholism have also been discussed as relevant behavioral addictions by scholars. Binge-Eating Disorder (BED) has been considered by some scholars to be one type of ICD, compulsive eating, or food addiction. The chapter of Eating Disorders in the *DSM-IV* includes Anorexia Nervosa, Bulimia Nervosa, and Eating Disorder Not Otherwise Specified (EDNOS). *DSM-IV* did not consider BED a free-standing diagnosis and classified it into EDNOS; BED was also included in Appendix of the *DSM-IV-TR* pending research.[19]

Although behavioral addiction is mainly classified in the category of ICDNEC in the *DSM-IV*, not all ICD or disorders with features of impulsivity are behavioral addictions.[20] In fact, the *DSM-IV* does not limit its ICD only to SRD and ICDNEC. It considers that the following disorders may also have characteristics of problems of impulse control: Paraphilias (under Sexual and Gender Identity Disorders in *DSM-IV*), Antisocial Personality Disorder, Conduct Disorder (under Disorders Usually First Diagnosed in Infancy, Childhood, or Adolescence in *DSM-IV*), Mood Disorders, and Schizophrenia.[21]

Definition of Impulsivity and Compulsivity

As mentioned earlier, one major characteristic of ICD is an individual's inability to resist a drive, temptation, or impulse to carry out an act that is detrimental to the individual or to others. *Impulsivity* can also be defined as "goal-directed behavior characterized by poor judgment in the attainment of rewards."[22] Furthermore, in many ICDs, compulsion—a repetitive, out-of-control engagement of a harmful behavior—is also part of the nature of the disease.[23] Although the American Psychiatric Association (APA) defined compulsions as repetitive behaviors or mental acts with an intention to prevent or decrease distress or anxiety, not to deliver gratification or pleasure, and although traditionally it may appear that impulsivity and *compulsivity* act toward opposite directions—impulsivity seeks pleasure despite possible harmful consequences, whereas compulsivity seeks safety and avoidance of harm—data have suggested that impulsivity and compulsivity may co-occur with the same psychiatric disorder such as an ICD[24, 25] or an OCD.[26, 27]

Possible Fundamental Reformulation and the *DSM-5*

There have been discussions of bringing together substance-related disorders and behavioral addiction disorders under one major category of ICD or addiction disorder, or reconceptualizing OCD—isolating it from anxiety disorder and making it an autonomous category of obsessive-compulsive spectrum disorder (OCSD)—to encompass both substance and multiple-behavioral addictions. There are both proponents and opponents of this expansion of addictive disorders. As of September 2012, the *DSM-5* work groups have proposed several reformations with respect to substance use disorder (SUD), gambling disorder, some ICDNECs, and other behavioral addictions, involving four newly named/revised chapters of "Substance Use and Addictive Disorders," "Obsessive-Compulsive and Related Disorders," "Feeding and Eating Disorders," and "Disruptive, Impulse Control, and Conduct Disorders," as well as the part of "Section III." (Note: The *DSM-5*-related contents were obtained before October of 2012, and they may or may not be subject to change before its final release in May of 2013.)

Substance Use and Addictive Disorders

Although the *DSM-IV* considers both substance-related disorders and some ICDs to possess similar qualities of impulsivity and compulsivity, it has separated them into two different classifications primarily because, compared with substance-related disorders, those ICDs in the ICDNEC category, except for pathological gambling, have not been systematically studied and clearly understood.[28] During 2010, the *DSM-5* Substance-Related Disorders work group proposed that SUD and pathological gambling be grouped under one new category, "Addiction and Related Disorders." The more recent name (as of September 2012) for the category is "Substance Use and Addictive Disorders."[29]

Although the *DSM-5* Substance-Related Disorders work group initially considered inclusion of Internet use disorder, Internet use disorder was later assigned into "Section III" for further research.[30] Like Internet use disorder, hypersexual disorder/sex addiction did not make it into this new category of Substance Use and Addictive Disorders or other new categories of Sexual Dysfunctions or Paraphilic Disorders, and instead, was recommended into the "Section III" pending research.[31]

Compulsive buying, another highly discussed behavioral addiction among the professionals and advocated for inclusion, was not being recommended by the *DSM-5* work groups into this new category. Some researchers suggest that compulsive buying shares many similarities with pathological gambling (the initial ego-syntonic urges were satisfied by shopping or gambling, but followed by guilt or shame) and may be considered as the female equivalent of pathological gambling—men tend to predominate among those with pathological gambling, whereas women tend to predominate among those with compulsive buying disorder.[32] It is not clear at this time about the *DSM-5* work groups' decision regarding compulsive buying.

In addition to keeping the diagnoses previously listed under the *DSM-IV* chapter of Substance-Related Disorders and taking in the Gambling Disorder from the *DSM-IV* chapter of ICDNEC, the newly proposed category "Substance Use and Addictive Disorders" a) reorganizes the order designations of the disorders in the category to be based on types of substance (for example, Alcohol-Related Disorders, with the subtypes of Alcohol Use Disorder, Alcohol Intoxication, Alcohol Withdrawal, Alcohol Induced Disorder Not Elsewhere Classified, Opioid-Related Disorders, with the subtypes of Opioid Use Disorder, Opioid Intoxication, Opioid Withdrawal, Opioid Induced Disorder Not Elsewhere Classified, and so on) instead of by types of diagnosis, such as use, intoxication, and withdrawal; b) combines substance dependence and substance abuse into one disorder; and c) consolidates Phencyclidine-Related Disorders into Hallucinogen-Related Disorders, simplifies the name "Sedative-, Hypnotic-, or Anxiolytic-Related Disorders" to just "Sedative/Hypnotic-Related Disorders," and unites all stimulant drugs, including amphetamines and cocaine, into one category of Stimulant-Related Disorders.[33]

Consolidating substance dependence and substance abuse into one unified SUD, as well as combining SUD and gambling disorder under one umbrella category of Substance Use and Addictive Disorders, has raised challenges. For example, Allen Frances, Chair of the *DSM-IV* Task Force, stated that the result of combining substance abuse and substance dependence would be that someone previously diagnosed with substance abuse in *DSM-IV* would now be diagnosed with Substance Use Disorder in *DSM-5*.[34] The title for the overall section so far appears to have been changed to "Substance Use and Addictive Disorders" from "the Addiction and Related Disorders."

Another issue is cutoff point or threshold. To be considered SUD positive under the *DSM-5*, a person needs to meet two or more of the eleven criteria, with zero or one criterion being no diagnosis; two to three criteria being mild SUD; four to five criteria being moderate SUD; and six or more criteria being severe SUD.[35] For Gambling Disorder (GD), the threshold is four or more of the nine criteria, with four or five criteria being mild GD; six or seven being moderate GD; and all or most all of nine criteria being severe GD.[36] Mitzner and colleagues suggest that perhaps the diagnostic threshold system applied to SUD can also be applied to GD since both are under the same umbrella category now. They suggest lowering the four criteria requirements to two so that subclinical gamblers can be identified.[37]

Bringing substance and nonsubstance behavioral addiction under one category has received some support from empirical research findings in the last decade. Evidence indicates that neuroadaptation (a change in brain circuitry) occurs not only when substance addiction is entailed, but also when nonsubstance behavioral addiction is involved.[38, 39, 40, 41] In other words, brain circuitry will be affected even in the absence of substance or pharmacological impact. Individuals with substance addiction and individuals with behavioral addiction may both experience a craving state prior to their substance consumption or behavior engagement, have weakened control over their problematic behavior, and continue such behavior despite negative and harmful consequences.[42]

Factors of family history and genetics, as well as comorbidity, also reveal the close relationship between substance-related disorders and ICDNEC, especially gambling disorder.[43, 44, 45] For example, Black et al.'s study indicated that 32.7 percent of the first-degree relatives of the individuals with pathological gambling disorder versus 14.8 percent of the control group had a lifetime history of substance use disorder.[46] Grant's clinical samples show that about 35–63 percent of the individuals with pathological gambling had a lifetime rate of substance use disorder, and the estimated lifetime rates of substance use disorder for individuals with kleptomania, compulsive sexual behavior, Internet addiction, compulsive buying, pathological skin picking, and intermittent explosive disorder, were 23–50 percent, 64 percent, 38 percent, 21–46 percent, 38 percent, and 48 percent, respectively.[47]

ICDNEC and substance-related disorders also benefit from similar psychosocial treatment methods. Many ICDs in the ICDNEC category, such as pathological gambling, kleptomania, compulsive buying, and compulsive sexual behavior, respond to the twelve-step approach, and others, such as pathological gambling, compulsive buying, trichotillomania, and pathological skin-picking, respond to cognitive behavioral therapy, as well as relapse prevention and lifestyle change strategies.[48] With respect to pharmacological treatment, although currently we do not have medications approved by the Food and Drug Administration (FDA) available for treatment of behavioral addiction, controlled or noncontrolled trials show that some medications effective for treatment of SUDs may also work for treatment of some behavioral addictions. For example, naltrexone, an opioid antagonist that proves to be effective with treatment of alcoholism and opioid dependence, has shown to also be beneficial in treating pathological gambling, kleptomania, and compulsive sexual behavior. However, effective treatment of these behavioral addictions requires a higher dosage of naltrexone than that for alcoholism. The mean dose is usually greater than 100 mg per day for the former whereas 50 mg or less per day for the latter, and the US FDA approves only 50 mg or less per day.[49]

Obsessive-Compulsive and Related Disorders

In 2010, the *DSM-5* Anxiety, Obsessive-Compulsive Spectrum, Posttraumatic, and Dissociative Disorders (AOCSPDD) work group proposed to have trichotillomania reclassified from the category of ICDNEC to the category of "Anxiety and Obsessive-Compulsive Spectrum Disorders." Later (as of September 2012), this work group proposed that Obsessive-Compulsive Disorders be an independent chapter from the Anxiety Disorders chapter. The new Obsessive-Compulsive and Related Disorders (OCRD) chapter will include not only the OCD previously listed in the *DSM-IV*, but also Body Dysmorphic Disorder (previously listed in the category of Somatoform Disorders in *DSM-IV*), Hoarding Disorder (not a formal diagnosis, but stated as one of the eight criteria for the Obsessive Compulsive Personality Disorder in the *DSM-IV*), Hair-Pulling Disorder (Trichotillomania, a formal diagnosis under ICDNEC in *DSM-IV*), Skin-Picking Disorder (not a formal diagnosis in *DSM-IV*), and so on.[50]

The *DSM-5* AOCSPDD work group further recommended, for Trichotillomania, replacing its old criterion B "An increasing sense of tension immediately before pulling out the hair or when attempting to resist the behavior" and criterion C "Pleasure, gratification, or relief when pulling out the hair" in the *DSM-IV* with the new criterion B "Repeated attempts to decrease or stop hair pulling" in *DSM-5*. The revision is based on the evidence that "patients with chronic hair-pulling may or may not meet *DSM-IV* criteria B or C, but do meet the proposed criterion."[51] Likewise, for Hoarding Disorder, the *DSM-5* work group chose the criterion "persistent difficulty discarding or parting with possessions, regardless of their actual value" over the criterion "the acquisition of and failure to discard a large number of possessions that appear to be useless or of limited value,"[52] and recommended the status of excessive acquisition or not to be a specifier. Although individuals with hoarding disorder excessively acquire things, not all individuals with hoarding problems engage in excessive acquisition, the *DSM-5* work group explained. On the other hand, information on whether a patient engages in excessive acquisition or not has implications for effective treatment, so the *DSM-5* work group recommended that it be a specifier instead of a criterion.[53] In both cases of the hair-pulling disorder and hoarding disorder, the *DSM-5* work group seems to downplay their pleasure-seeking or ego-syntonic features, and thus make it even more reasonable to categorize them under the category of "Obsessive-Compulsive and Related Disorders."

Also, the work group considers the word "mania" inappropriate for trichotillomania disorder and recommends "hair-pulling disorder" instead but, to avoid confusion, suggesting the use of "hair-pulling disorder (trichotillomania)."[54] Because of the significant clinical similarities between skin-picking disorder and hair-pulling disorder, the diagnosis criteria for each mirror the other.[55]

Grouping ICDs under the umbrella of Obsessive-Compulsive Spectrum Disorder (OCSD) has been considered by the psychiatric community since the 1990s. In 2006, a conference targeting OCSD was convened to examine disorders that should be included in the category of OCSD. Among them are OCD, obsessive-compulsive personality disorder, Tourette's syndrome (and other tic disorders), autism, eating disorders, ICDs, and substance addictions.[56, 57] One reason for suggesting that ICD be grouped under OCSD is that scholars have found that ICD, like OCD, possesses compulsive characteristics—that is, a repetitive engagement in the behavior[58] that causes the behavior to continue over time.[59]

However, some scholars pointed out that OCD and ICD have a major difference, in that OCD involves the ego-dystonic nature (avoiding harm) whereas ICD has the ego-syntonic nature (seeking pleasure).[60] Explanations have been proposed to counteract this criticism. For example, a pathological gambler may initially gamble to seek pleasure (ego-syntonic), later realize the negative consequences involved, and then experience irritability when attempting to stop or cut down the gambling, and consequently struggle with continuing gambling. The individual is now primarily seeking stress reduction or anxiety alleviation rather than pleasure, and the urge has become more ego-dystonic than ego-syntonic.[61]

Another insight is that ICD may be a group with heterogeneous disorders and that some ICDs may be closer to OCD than other ICDs. For example, Grant et al. found that pathological skin-picking and nail-biting were more prevalent than other ICDs among participants with OCD.[62] Bienvenu et al. also found that although their OCD group tended to have a higher rate of "grooming disorders" (trichotillomania, pathological nail-biting, and pathological skin-picking) than their non-OCD group, there was no significant difference with respect to other ICDs (e.g., pathological gambling, pyromania, and kleptomania) between the OCD and non-OCD groups.[63] This may suggest that trichotillomania, pathological nail-biting, and pathological skin-picking resemble OCD more than other ICDs do.

Feeding and Eating Disorders

The *DSM-5* Eating Disorders work group has recommended promotion of binge-eating disorder (BED) from a disorder that had no distinct code, was under the "Eating Disorder Not Otherwise Specified" of the category of Eating Disorders in *DSM-IV*, and was included in the Appendix for further study in the *DSM-IV-TR*, to an independent and formal diagnosis, along with Anorexia Nervosa and Bulimia Nervosa in the category of Eating Disorders.[64] The revision is based on strong empirical findings that binge-eating disorder can be meaningfully differentiated from other eating disorders and that individuals with BED show a significant level of eating-disorder psychopathology, psychiatric comorbidity, and impairment in life quality that is similar to the level experienced by individuals with other eating disorder diagnoses.[65, 66]

The work group also recommended renaming the category from "Eating Disorders" to "Feeding and Eating Disorders." The new category will include not only the eating disorders listed in the *DSM-IV*, but also the feeding disorders, such as Pica and Rumination Disorder, that were previously listed under the category of Disorders Usually First Diagnosed in Infancy, Childhood, or Adolescence in *DSM-IV*.[67]

Disruptive, Impulse Control, and Conduct Disorders

The *DSM-5* ADHD and Disruptive Behavior Disorders work group and other work groups have proposed breaking the chapter of "Disorders Usually First Diagnosed in Infancy, Childhood, or Adolescence" in the *DSM-IV-TR* and reassigning its various diagnoses into several other newly developed or revised categories in *DSM-5*. Among the new categories are Neurodevelopmental Disorders (including Autism Spectrum Disorders, Attention Deficit Hyperactivity Disorders, and so on),[68] Feeding and Eating Disorder (for example, Pica, Rumination Disorder, and so on),[69] and "Disruptive, Impulse Control, and Conduct Disorders."[70]

The new category of Disruptive, Impulse Control, and Conduct Disorders contains Oppositional Defiant Disorder, Conduct Disorder, Dyssocial Personality Disorder (Antisocial Personality Disorder), and the Intermittent Explosive Disorder, which was previously under the *DSM-IV* ICDNEC. The *DSM-5* work group proposed six diagnosis criteria for the Intermittent Explosive Disorder, to which the *DSM-IV* assigned only three criteria previously. One of the new criterion is "chronological age is at least eighteen years (or equivalent developmental level)."[71]

"Section III"

"Section III" of the *DSM-5* includes disorders that require further research before they can be considered free-standing diagnoses and perhaps be categorized in future *DSM*s. Currently, at the time of this writing—September of 2012—four substance- and addictive-related disorders were recommended by the *DSM-5* work groups to be added to "Section III." They are Neurobehavioral Disorder Associated with Prenatal Alcohol Exposure, Caffeine Use Disorder, Hypersexual Disorder (belonging to the ICDNOS of the ICDNEC or a sexual disorder, NOS in *DSM-IV*, conceptualized under the category of Paraphilic Disorders or the category of Sexual Dysfunctions in *DSM-5*),[72] and Internet Use Disorder (belonging to the ICDNOS of the ICDNEC in *DSM-IV*, and conceptualized under Substance Use and Addictive Disorders in *DSM-5*).[73] (In December of 2012, the American Psychiatric Association decided not to include Hypersexual Disorder in Sections III or II.)

Why We Should Learn About Behavioral Addiction

Grouping ICDNEC and the SRD under one umbrella of Addiction and Related Disorders or grouping Impulse-Control Disorder with OCD and other disorders under one umbrella of Obsessive Compulsive Spectrum Disorders is controversial and may each involve advantages and disadvantages. Regardless of whether those disorders are reorganized, practitioners and researchers, especially those who work with substance-abusing clients, should be prepared with the knowledge and skills to understand and effectively help clients with behavioral addiction.

There are four reasons for this. First, like substance addiction, nonsubstance behavioral addictions take place in both the general population and the psychiatric clinical population, and cause distress and impairment in the addicted person. Second, research has indicated that although in a less direct and less powerful way, compared with substance addiction, behavioral addiction can similarly affect a person's brain circuitry, creating salience, learning and reinforcing, a lower inhibition, and a drive to "go," executing the harmful behavior. Third, the advancement of technology may facilitate new forms of behavioral addiction (e.g., compulsive Internet use and online video games) or create newer forms of old behavioral addictions (e.g., Internet pornography addiction and online gambling). The new ethos of an ever-changing society may also precipitate new forms of behavioral addictions; for example, widespread media promotion of consumerism, which encourages spending, which in turn plants seeds of compulsive spending among certain at-risk populations. Fourth, behavioral addictions usually co-occur with substance addiction and/or other major psychiatric disorders (e.g., depression, bipolar disorders, ADHD, OCD). To effectively help clients who have a psychiatric diagnosis with co-occurring disorders, it is critical that clinicians be equipped with knowledge and skills with respect to all the related, comorbid disorders, including behavioral addiction. The following elaborates on these four reasons.

Reason 1: Prevalence and consequences

Behavioral addictions and impulse control disorders occur in the general population and are overrepresented in the clinical population with psychiatric disorders; however, they tend to be underappreciated, underdiagnosed, and understudied.[74] While looking for the prevalence of behavioral addictions among the general population, we were able to locate only the National Comorbidity Survey Replication (NCS-R) study. Although NCS-R provides estimates of "impulse control disorders" (ICD), it defines ICD somewhat differently when compared with the ICDs or other behavioral addictions in other studies. ICDs in NCS-R include the oppositional defiant disorder, conduct disorder, attention-deficit/hyperactivity disorder, and intermittent explosive disorder.[75] The results of NCS-R showed that 8.9 percent of the US general population has a current ICD and 24.8 percent has a lifetime history of ICD.[76] According to Grant et al.'s study, 30.9 percent of the adult psychiatric populations (admission diagnoses included mood disorder, substance use disorder, anxiety disorder, psychotic disorder, etc.) have at least one current ICD, with compulsive buying being most common, followed by kleptomania and pathological gambling, and 32.8 percent have at least one lifetime ICD.[77] Müller and colleagues found that 18.8 percent of the psychiatric inpatients (a European sample) have a current ICD, with pathological skin-picking being most common, followed by compulsive buying and intermittent explosive disorder, and 23.5 percent have a lifetime ICD.[78]

With inconsistent and differing diagnostic criteria, screening, and assessment tools adopted by researchers and clinicians, as well as the varying availability of gambling opportunities, the estimated rates of pathological gambling varied. According to Petry's review, if measured by the South Oaks Gambling Screen (SOGS), the rates in the United States are 1.6–4.0

percent, and in other countries, 0.8–6.0 percent; if measured by *DSM-IV*-based scales, the rates in the United States are 0.4–2.0 percent.[79] The estimated rates of Internet addiction appear to vary even more widely than those of pathological gambling. Weinstein and Lejoyeux's review shows that the rates are about 0.3–6 percent in the US general population, 2.4–6.44 percent in two provinces in China, 17.9 percent in a study on Taiwanese university freshmen, and 18.3 percent in a study on British students.[80] It appears that no systematic studies have been done on the prevalence rates of sexual addiction among the general population using standardized diagnostic criteria, but the rates in the United States are estimated to be 3–6 percent.[81] The rates may be higher among some specific groups; for example, one study shows that significantly more incarcerated sexual offenders meet the threshold of sexual addiction than their community participants (35 percent versus 12.5 percent).[82]

For compulsive buying, Koran and colleagues' survey[83] shows an estimated rate of 5.8 percent among the US general population; however, the rates are much higher among some specific groups, ranging from 17.7 percent among shoppers of a women's clothing Internet retailer to 32.5 percent found among women customers at a Parisian department store.[84] According to the NCS-R survey, the estimated lifetime history prevalence of binge eating disorder measured by the *DSM-IV* criteria is 2.8 percent for the US general population (3.5 percent for women and 2.0 percent for men) and the estimated current (twelve month) prevalence is 1.2 percent (1.6 percent for women and 0.8 percent for men).[85] Binge eating disorder is more prevalent among severely obese populations who seek treatment; the rate is 25–30 percent among those who participate in weight control programs and 70 percent among Overeaters Anonymous (OA) members.[86, 87]

It would be interesting to compare the prevalence rates of substance use disorders with those of behavioral addictions. The 2010 National Survey on Drug Use and Health results show that the estimated rate of past-year substance dependence or abuse among age twelve or older Americans is 8.7 percent, and the rates for "alcohol dependence or abuse" and for "illicit drug dependence or abuse" are 7.0 percent and 2.8 percent, respectively.[88] Although the prevalence rates of substance dependence or abuse may appear to be greater than those of the behavioral addictions listed above, the gap is not as wide as previously perceived, especially if we compare the behavioral addictions with the illicit-drug dependence or abuse.

Although substance addiction may have a stronger effect on the human brain than behavioral addiction owing to its pharmacological implications, it is a myth that behavioral addiction causes less harmful consequences than substance addiction. Behavioral addiction and impulse control disorders may result in low self-esteem, depression, anxiety, trauma, and distress.[89] It may lead to conflicted marital and family or other interpersonal relationships, poor academic or job performance, substance abuse, and social/legal problems. Some behavioral addictions may even be linked to suicide[90] or homicide. For example, in 2007, a seventeen-year-old Ohio teenage boy killed his mother and injured his father because they removed his computer video game. The father told the judge that his son does not understand why he committed such terrible behavior. The judge said the boy's obsession with the video game may have led him to believe that "death wasn't real," just like those creatures in the game. News in Taiwan recently reported such a case: A twenty-eight-year-old woman murdered her own mother, her mother-in-law, and her husband in order to benefit from their life insurance to pay the huge debt she had incurred from her gambling addiction.

Reason 2: Brain effects

The National Institute on Drug Abuse (NIDA) and other scientists' brain disease theory suggests that addiction is a brain disease resulting from the interaction among salience/reward, learning/memory/conditioning, and a lowering inhibition/control.

Scientists suggest that wherever there is a reward sensed by the brain regions of *nucleus accumbens* and *ventral tegmental area* (VTA) because of ingestion of AOD or due to certain behaviors or acts, there is a sense of salience produced with respect to AOD or those behaviors and acts. Such a sense of salience will be remembered by the person or reinforced through the function of memory/learning or conditioning executed by the brain regions of the *amygdala* and the hippocampus. Furthermore, exposure to AOD or other rewarding experiences may weaken a person's inhibitory and control capacity, which is executed by the brain regions of anterior cingulate gyrus and *prefrontal cortex*. Together, all three components will create a huge motivation and drive to prompt the person to "go" ahead, consuming AOD or performing the rewarding behaviors or acts repeatedly and compulsively in spite of facing negative consequences caused by those rewarding substances or behaviors.[91]

A person can potentially become addicted to almost anything in the world, as long as that particular thing can provide reward to the person. In fact, scholars stated that "life is a series of addictions," involving breathing, eating, drinking, and having sex, and "without them we die."[92] Researchers pointed out that the human brain has a "built-in rewarding system" that reinforces and sustains our basic drive, so that basic human needs for survival and continuation of the human species—such as feeding, fight/flight, reproduction, parenting, and so on—can be fulfilled. Both substance addiction and behavioral addiction, however, may disturb the natural rewarding drive and process that sustains humans' normal survival mechanism, misdirect the drive to pursue harmful actions, and leave little energy for more constructive facets of life.[93] Drugs can increase brain dopamine up to two to ten times stronger than natural rewards.[94]

Although substance addiction may have a more direct and powerful effect on the human brain than nonsubstance behavioral addiction because substances may bind with brain receptors and create pharmacological effects directly on brain circuits, the nonsubstance behavioral addiction (e.g., pathological gambling, compulsive shopping, sex, eating, and/ or Internet use) may also have an effect on the human brain and generate a similar path of effect.[95, 96] Olsen's literature review reveals that "like substance addictions, nondrug addictions manifest in similar psychological and behavioral patterns, including craving, impaired control over the behavior, tolerance, withdrawal, and high rates of relapse. Similarities between drugs and nondrug rewards can also be seen physiologically. Functional neuroimaging studies in humans have shown that gambling, shopping, orgasm, playing video games, and the sight of appetizing food, activate many of the same brain regions (i.e., the mesocorticolimbic system and extended amygdala) as drugs of abuse."[97]

The discovery of the shared brain vulnerabilities between substance and nonsubstance addiction not only direct us to recast addiction (e.g., placing substance use disorder and gambling disorder in the same category rather than separating them), but also can stimulate new findings of crossover pharmacotherapies and benefit both substance and nonsubstance addictions.[98]

Reason 3: Our ever-changing society

Although the advances of technology and its effect on our society overall as well as a changing social climate and lifestyles may enhance the quality of human life, they may also precipitate problems and pathologies. The public health model suggests that in order for a disease to occur, there must be an agent, an at-risk host, and a disease-enabling environment. The constantly emerging new technology and culture may unintentionally create new forms of old addictions, generate a new agent, or facilitate an environment that triggers diseases.

One example is compulsive shopping, which is not a newly identified disorder but was termed "oniomania" by Kraepelin in 1915.[99] Although individuals with low self-esteem or depression may be more prone to compulsive shopping, the environment and culture may contribute further to the vulnerability. Citing various authors, Lee and Mysyk stated that one explanation for compulsive buying is that television, including game shows and soap operas, and print commercials and other media frequently cultivate a material attitude, instill a desire to purchase, and glorify luxurious spending among the general population, regardless of an individual's gender and socioeconomic status.[100] Easy access to credit further perpetuates out-of-control shopping behaviors among certain at-risk populations. Dittmar and Drury quoted one compulsive buyer who stated that "it never feels like you're actually spending money if you use credit cards."[101] Another compulsive buyer said, "Buying something and charging it was like getting it for free with no future accounting or consequence."[102] Consumerism also encourages "consumption to excess." It is not uncommon for grocery or department stores to post signs like, "Buy two and get the second one free," and for fast-food restaurants to increase the size or content of their servings, just to entice customers and to compete with peer stores.

Compulsive video game playing or Internet use disorder is another example. Computers and the Internet may not only lead to excessive use because of their pure rewarding effects like a sense of accomplishment and social interactions, but also can become the new agents or tools for multiple old obsessions. For example, compulsive sex may be in the form of Internet pornography or cybersex and pathological gambling may take place on the Internet. Internet pornography has become the most profitable category of the various Internet activities, offering a new, alluring outlet to fulfill their addiction not only for individuals with sex addiction problems, but also for some at-risk individuals who have never experienced sex addiction problems. Internet pornography may hook them once they bump into it.[103] Young presented a statement by a fifty-two-year-old lawyer who was married for thirty-five years: "I wasn't the kind of man to look at pornography . . . . One night while working late, I stumbled onto an adult website. Soon after, I was completely hooked. Every time I felt stressed with another deadline at work, I relaxed by looking at porn sites . . . I started to miss meetings, miss important deadlines. I tried to stop. I'd quit for a while, and then the process would start all over again. I lost my job, my marriage, everything that was important to me."[104]

Likewise, the "disease-enabling environment" concept applies to the issue of obesity or compulsive-eating/overeating behavior. Volkow and Wise stated that ". . . genes that were favored under conditions of food scarcity have become a liability in societies where high-energy, highly refined foods are prevalent and readily affordable."[105] They suggest that the recent rise in the rate of obesity has a lot to do with the dramatically increased accessibility of seductive foods (e.g., high-carbohydrate, high-fat, and low-cost) and the growing availability of vending machines, fast-food restaurants, and convenience stores, as the genome has not changed much.[106]

Reason 4: Co-occurrence

Finally, the high co-occurring rate of behavioral addiction with other psychiatric disorders (e.g., substance addiction, depression, bipolar disorders, eating disorders, ADHD, OCD, and so on) points to the importance for practitioners and students in the field of mental health in general, and substance abuse treatment in particular, to be equipped with knowledge and skills with respect to behavioral addiction and its treatment. For example, the results of the National Epidemiologic Survey on Alcohol and Related Conditions show that the rates of lifetime history of alcohol use disorder, drug use disorder, mood disorder, anxiety disorder, and personality disorder among individuals with lifetime history of pathological gambling were 73.2 percent, 38.1 percent, 49.6 percent, 41.3 percent, and 60.8 percent, respectively.[107] Nicola and colleagues found that 33 percent of the bipolar patients versus 13 percent of the healthy controls in their study presented at least one behavioral addiction (for example, pathological gambling, compulsive buying, sexual and work addictions).[108] The study of Yen and colleagues shows an association between Internet addiction and symptoms of ADHD, depression, and social phobia among adolescents.[109]

The Center for Substance Abuse Treatment (CSAT) recently called for increased attention to the co-occurring phenomenon of an independent mental disorder (e.g., bipolar disorders or schizophrenia) and an independent substance-use disorder (e.g., alcohol dependence).[110] Both practitioners and researchers have become aware that treating one disorder without treating the other proves ineffective in treating either. The same applies to behavioral addiction. To take Internet addiction as an example, adolescents (or adults) may use the Internet to help cope with their emotional stress or psychiatric disorders such as depression; it would be less effective to treat Internet addiction without intervening in the psychiatric disorders of the individuals. Likewise, addictive or compulsive Internet use provides ineffective coping and generates more difficulty in real life, and therefore, if not addressed, may further deteriorate a person's psychiatric disorder(s) and compromise the person's treatment.[111] In addition, Martin and Petry suggest that "treatment outcome for each drive disorder improves if all co-occurring out-of-control behaviors are addressed, as relapse in one behavioral realm often triggers the reemergence of co-occurring pathological behaviors."[112]

Conclusion

The phenomenon of behavior addiction was identified at least a century ago, but began to emerge only in the past decades. Old, new, and new forms of old behavior addictions have been heightened by enormous social, technological, and cultural changes. The *DSM-5*, which is scheduled for release in May of 2013, has currently recommended placing both substance use disorders and gambling disorder under the same classification of "Substance Use and Addictive Disorders." The *DSM-5* also has so far proposed inclusion of "Internet Use Gaming Disorder" in

"Section III," pending research before it can be considered for promotion to become a formal diagnosis. Although *DSM-5* work groups have strived for a balance between being creative and being conservative in updating the *DSM*, they received many criticisms, one being the possibility of diagnostic inflation and the creation of false epidemics. Since most behavior addictions are extensions of normal human needs, it is challenging to draw a line between a personal lifestyle and a psychiatric pathology. Nonetheless, the media are reporting more and more tragedies related to addictive behavior problems and clinicians are seeing more and more clients and their significant others seeking help for out-of-control, addictive behavior problems. Research data further indicate the close relationship and similarities between substance and behavior addictions. The strong scientific evidence of the occurrence of behavioral addictions with other major, well-established psychiatric diagnoses such as depression, anxiety, bipolar, ADHD, and substance use disorder further suggests the importance for mental health professionals to screen for and treat behavior addiction problems in addition to other psychiatric diagnoses among their clients. Although many treatment modalities and approaches for substance use disorders can be adapted for treatment of behavior addiction, more research is needed to disentangle the complicated relationships among behavior addiction, substance addiction, impulse-control disorder, and obsessive-compulsive disorder, because such research can help develop best practices, both psychosocial and pharmacological, for the treatment of behavior addictions.

2

The Brain and Addiction

Lesley Dickson, MD

Much has been learned in the recent past about addiction to substances, which is referred to as Substance Use Disorders in *DSM-IV*-TR.[1] But the understanding of what is behavioral addiction, what causes it to develop, and what maintains such an addiction has lagged. This is at least partly due to the ease of studying the effects of drugs in animal models and the fact that drugs are chemicals and chemicals cause chemical changes by altering neurotransmitters in brains and other parts of the body. However, it has become more apparent that learning models must also be developed to explain the fact that addiction and related behaviors persist even without the presence of the drugs themselves. These learning models may be particularly useful in understanding behavioral addiction, but one should also consider that the endogenous neurotransmitters are at play in these repetitive and potentially destructive behaviors. Therefore, it is useful to review what is known about how substances are believed to cause addiction and then try to extend that knowledge to nonsubstance or behavioral addiction.

How Do People Become Addicted?

Basic understanding of human and animal behavior has led to the concept that individuals will seek to experience pleasure and avoid pain or other forms of displeasure. While Freud and other theorists have described behaviors such as the compulsions that are lacking in pleasure but are sought after in certain circumstances, generally individuals will try to create or maintain situations where pleasure outweighs displeasure. It is the pleasure feeling that leads to the concept of reward and then the likelihood that the individual will seek to re-experience that feeling—and in addiction, to such a frequency of seeking that experience that the individual continues to do so in spite of multiple negative consequences.

Basic Neuroscience

The location of the pleasure and reward experience is the brain, which is organized into functional areas, nuclei, and circuits. Functions such as thought, memory, and emotion occur through complicated circuits between areas and nuclei, and therefore, interruptions of various points of a circuit can lead to psychiatric symptoms.[2] The brain consists of nerve cells or *neurons*. These neurons have a cell body with a nucleus, cytoplasm, and membranes with extensions known as *dendrites* and *axons*. The dendrites carry information in the form of an electrical impulse to the cell body and axons carry information away from the cell body and to other neurons. The neuron contains the filamentous components of microtubules, neurofilaments, and actin, which make up the cell's skeleton and perform many structural duties, including movement of molecules and formation of *synapses*.

Neurons communicate with each other by the release of molecules into the small space between their cell membranes known as the *synaptic cleft* with the presynaptic cell membrane, the synaptic cleft, and the postsynaptic membrane making up the synapse. These molecules are known as *neurotransmitters* and once released, usually following the arrival of an electrical impulse or action potential, can bind to specific sites known as *receptors* on the next neuron. The binding of a neurotransmitter to a receptor can increase or decrease the likelihood of an electrical transmission down the axon of the neuron and also lead to chemical changes within the neuron. The electrical transmission can then cause another release of neurotransmitters to other neurons or *effector cells,* such as motor fibers, allowing neurons to communicate rapidly with each other and other organs of the body.[3, 4]

Neurotransmitters and Receptors

Many naturally occurring or endogenous neurotransmitters have been identified and most can be localized to specific regions of the brain while a few, such as glutamate and GABA, are widespread. Additionally, neurotransmitters generally have fairly specific functions determined by their chemical composition and the receptors to which they bind. Neurotransmitters are of two types—small molecules, such as dopamine and serotonin and larger *neuropeptides*, such as the endorphins and some of the hormones. The small molecule neurotransmitters are stored in membrane-surrounded vesicles within the neuron and are released when an action potential arrives. This action causes an influx of calcium leading to the vesicle membrane fusing with the cell membrane at the presynaptic area and release of the neurotransmitter into the synaptic cleft. Receptors are proteins embedded in the cell membranes of neurons and when they are activated by the binding of a specific neurotransmitter, can cause chemical changes within the neuron that ultimately may lead to some long-lasting alterations in the neuron. Memory and learned behavior are thought to result from these long-standing chemical changes.

The action of neurotransmitters can be controlled in many ways by neurons, and these operations are frequently the site of the action of many drugs of abuse as well as medications.

Neurotransmitter levels in the synapse determine the amount available for receptor binding and therefore can be modified by several mechanisms. The amount of transmitter available can vary due to the control of its synthesis within the neuron. Packaging into vesicles and release from the vesicles into the synaptic cleft can be altered such as seen with the amphetamines, which increase dopamine release. While neurotransmitters may diffuse away from the synaptic cleft, they are frequently removed back into the originating neuron from the synapse via a transporter molecule by a process known as *reuptake*. Blocking of reuptake of the neurotransmitters dopamine and serotonin is the main action of cocaine and the intended effect of medications such as antidepressants. Neurotransmitters can be metabolically broken down in the synapse as seen in the action of acetylcholinesterase on acetylcholine, which has led to the use of inhibitors of the enzyme to increase acetylcholine levels in Alzheimer's disease. Meanwhile, the postsynaptic neuron can control the response to the neurotransmitter by altering the number of receptors and the configuration of the receptor in the cell membrane.[5]

Postsynaptic Receptors

There are two types of receptors, *ionotropic* and *metabotropic*.[6] The ionotropic receptors are rapid and linked to ion channels that undergo a conformational change after binding to a neurotransmitter that opens the channel and either leads to depolarization and propagation of an action potential or hyperpolarization, which inhibits an action potential. The excitatory neurotransmitter is *glutamate* and there are two glutamate receptors, the NMDA and the non-NMDA receptors, AMPA and *kainate* receptors. The NMDA receptor plus glutamate allows calcium (Ca^{2+}) to enter and generate an action potential and is also involved in new synapse formation, learning, memory, and cell death when glutamate levels are high. Similar functions are provided by the non-NMDA receptors but also appear to include long-term potentiation, which is involved in anxiety states. Alcohol is thought to exert some of its effects on the AMPA receptors by causing *upregulation* of the receptor after long-term use.[7]

GABA and its receptors perform the major inhibitory functions of the brain. $GABA_A$ receptors are ionotropic receptors that allow chloride (Cl^-) influx and therefore inhibit electrical impulses by hyperpolarization of the cell membrane. $GABA_A$ receptors are targets of drugs such as benzodiazepines, which bind to a recognition site and mediate their sedating and anxiolytic effects, unfortunately leading to a significant addiction problem of these legal and useful prescription drugs.[8]

Metabotropic receptors such as those for serotonin and dopamine mediate long-term effects and generally are not linked to ion channels.[9] Rather, they are linked to intracellular processes including G proteins that are activated by binding to GTP and then couple with second messengers. This action can then lead to enzymatic reactions such as phosphorylation of proteins that mediates activation or inactivation of these proteins potentially changing membrane channels, altering cytoskeletal elements, and initiating gene transcription by migrating to the cell nucleus. Gene transcription ultimately results in synthesis of new proteins, particularly those involved in increasing the strength of synaptic connections and thus reinforcing neural pathways involved in learning.

Dopamine

The neurotransmitter that has been shown to most associate with the experience of pleasure is dopamine, abbreviated as DA.[10] The cell bodies of the neurons that make DA are located in the midbrain in two small areas known as the *substantia nigra* (SN) and the ventral tegmental area (VTA). The VTA DA-containing neurons project to several regions of the brain, including the areas known as the *nucleus accumbens* (NAcc), the amygdalae, and the prefrontal cortex. SN neurons connect with the *basal ganglia*, an area that is important in movement. The loss of these neurons leads to Parkinson's disease, which is frequently treated with dopamine replacement.

The most direct connection of the DA neurons to a substance introduced from the outside is that of cocaine. Cocaine blocks the reuptake of DA, leading to increased amounts in the synapse and a rapid onset of a feeling of intense pleasure or euphoria. Amphetamines also increase the amount of DA in the synapse by increasing the release into the synapse. Another phenomenon is desensitization that occurs after postsynaptic DA receptors have been repeatedly stimulated and the amount of DA receptors is decreased, thus leading to less sensitivity to DA, also known as *down-regulation* or neuronal tolerance. This group of "stimulants" has been most effectively studied and their mechanisms well documented. The stimulants produce addiction rapidly in both animal models and humans and the long-term effects of cravings and cue-induced responses are serving as models for understanding the learning process and the formation of memory.

Other Neurotransmitters

Several other important neurotransmitters and their receptors have been associated with the drugs of abuse.[11] The endorphins that bind to specific opiate receptors related to the experience of pain and relaxation are easily substituted by the highly addictive opioid drugs such as heroin, morphine, and many prescribed pain medications. GABA and glutamate are *amino acids*, which act as neurotransmitters and are widespread with GABA as the major inhibitory neurotransmitter and glutamate the major excitatory one. Many of the sedating drugs such as the benzodiazepines work via GABA receptors, while alcohol has an effect on the glutamate system. Serotonin is a neurotransmitter that is important in mood disorders, impulsivity, and aggression and modifying its activity has been important in the treatment of depression by drugs that block reuptake in the synapse while LSD blocks serotonin receptors and cocaine can increase its concentration by reuptake blocking. *Norepinephrine* (NE), sometimes referred to as noradrenaline, is synthesized in cells located in the *nucleus coeruleus* of the *pons* and functions to regulate arousal, dreaming, and moods while also functioning as a hormone that increases blood pressure and heart rate under conditions of stress. Acetylcholine is an important neurotransmitter in both the brain and the rest of the body as it excites other neurons, as well as muscles, tissues, and glands. Nicotine, the most common drug of abuse, binds to nicotinic acetylcholine receptors in the brain resulting in one of the most pervasive and difficult to treat addictions. Finally, the more recently discovered *endocannabinoids* bind to the receptors that also bind the active ingredient in marijuana, THC. The prevailing thought has been that while all the exogenously introduced drugs will interact with specific receptors, the actions they initiate will ultimately lead to neurons that make contact with DA containing neurons and the drug of abuse therefore provokes an increase in dopamine and the feeling of pleasure and reward. However, Koob and Le Moal point out that dopamine is not necessarily required for the reinforcing effects of some of the nonstimulant drugs of abuse or some natural or nondrug rewards thus suggesting the DA schema will need to be expanded.[12]

Neural Circuits

The main reward pathway in the brain is considered to be the *mesolimbic dopamine system* (MDS), which consists of the dopamine neurons projecting forward from the VTA to the nucleus accumbens, the amygdalae, the *anterior cingulate cortex*, and the frontal and prefrontal cortex. Much of this system is part of the *subcortical* brain with actions taking place out of consciousness and thus the development of drug dependence is mostly outside conscious awareness.[13] Also, the effects of drugs on the projections to the frontal lobes are what probably lead to the loss of control over drug use through a reduction of cortical decision making. This decrease in function in the prefrontal and cingulated cortex can be demonstrated by fMRI studies where cocaine addicts and those with pathological gambling showed decreased activity in response to viewing activity-specific videotapes.[14]

Other important circuits in the MDS are the glutamate neurons that project from the prefrontal cortex to the NAcc and the VTA and the GABA neurons projecting from the NAcc to the prefrontal cortex. There are also opioid *interneurons*, which are short interconnections that can affect the GABA neuronal actions and the NE neurons originating in the *locus coeruleus*. Serotonin neurons from the *raphe nucleus* also project to the VTA and NAcc.[15] Thus most of the drugs of abuse interact with this system, and the development of medications to treat drug abuse is often aimed at effecting change at one or more of these connections.

As the circuits of the MDS have been established, research tools have been developed to understand their function. PET scanning and fMRI can look at these areas of the brain and demonstrate differences between control subjects and individuals who are under the influence of drugs or who have a long history of drug use. In animal models, electrical stimulation and ablation techniques can determine the function of specific cells and their connections. Drugs have been developed that can block or stimulate neurotransmission at specific receptor sites in animals that have been trained to seek out and self-dispense drugs of abuse, whereby models of substance abuse are created. From these models, researchers are now identifying the mechanisms that maintain the desire for a drug, i.e., craving, and the return to drug use after years of abstinence even when there is a lack of the drug in the environment. These learning models may then aid in explaining the addictive behaviors that do not involve substances but clearly have a reward to the individual engaging in them.

Neuroplasticity, Learning, and Memory

Much of what maintains an individual's use of several of the drugs of abuse in spite of negative consequences is the physical and psychological discomfort that occurs when the drug is withdrawn. This is frequently intense, particularly with the opioids, and can be deadly in the case of alcohol. Withdrawal symptoms are generally the opposite of intoxication symptoms and can mostly be explained by the physiological responses due to the changes in the affected neurotransmitter levels or the postsynaptic receptors' adjustments to the absence of the drug. Since the physiological adjustment is accomplished over a period of days, there must be long-lasting changes that maintain the addiction and these are in the memory functions of the brain.

Learning and memory take place at the synapses via short- and long-term changes. As described earlier, neurotransmitters are released in response to stimuli from the environment with drugs of abuse being more powerful than other stimuli, such as physiological drives, sensory input, or pleasurable activities such as exercise.[16] The neurotransmitters bind to specific postsynaptic receptors and activate second messenger systems that lead to many intracellular changes and remodeling and strengthening of the synaptic connections.[17, 18] The hippocampus is the primary location for encoding memory, and with high-frequency stimulation there is long-term potentiation (LTP), which may last for weeks at the synaptic connections, primarily via NMDA and AMPA receptors. Early LTP is short-acting and does not require protein synthesis while late LTP, lasting several hours or more, does involve gene transcription and protein translation and requires dopamine binding at D_1 receptors. Late LTP includes the permanent alterations of synapses involved in learning and memory and when seen under the microscope, consists of increased density of the spiny processes of the dendrites, suggesting an increased number of synapses at these important connections.

Kalivas and Volkow propose that end-stage addiction, described as such an intense desire to use the drug of choice that there is almost total loss of control and lack of interest in other activities, results from cellular adaptations in the prefrontal cortex neurons and their projections to the nucleus accumbens.[19] The prefrontal cortex regulates the amount of importance or salience that is attached to a stimulus and then determines the intensity of the responsive behavior. The glutamate projections from the prefrontal cortex impact the NAcc, the amygdala (important in emotional response and the appreciation of environmental and interoceptive stressors), and the thalamus. The GABA neurons of the NAcc then project to the *ventral pallidum*, which is critical for motivated behavior. Dopamine projections from the VTA release DA into this circuit and serve to alert the organism of novel and salient stimuli leading to learning, as well as alerting the organism of pending appearance of a familiar and motivationally relevant event based on these learned associations. Everitt and Robbins add that stimuli in the environment that are closely associated in time and space to the drug use also develop "incentive salience" through Pavlovian-type conditioning and then become cues for relapse.[20] Wise, one of the earliest to describe the dopamine reward hypothesis has added that it is the receipt of reward predictors (promise of reward) that produces the highest arousal and that these rewards are conditioned rewards from previous learning.[21] Wise includes the normal pleasures of life in addition to the drugs of abuse and electrical stimulation as reward predictors and suggests how the non-drug related addictions may develop.[22]

3

Gambling Addiction

Larry Ashley, EdS, LCADC, CPGC

Karmen K. Boehlke, MS

Chance is an intrinsic feature of life; consequently, gambling appeals to the inherent risk-taking nature of human beings. A cursory review through the archives of gambling literature leaves little doubt that gambling and games of change have been popular activities for human beings throughout the history of humankind. For example, dice were found in an Egyptian tomb that dated to approximately 3,000 BC. A gaming board was cut into the steps of the Acropolis at Athens.[1]

Gambling in North America preceded the founding of the United States. When European settlers and explorers arrived on the Atlantic seaboard in the sixteenth and seventeenth centuries, they encountered native tribes that had well-established systems of wagering. For example, early explorers in New York witnessed members of the Onondaga tribe placing bets on the role of stone dice.[2]

However, gambling in the New World was not limited solely to native cultures. Historical reports claim that George Washington purchased the first lottery ticket that financed the colony of Virginia's development.[3] Additionally, lotteries also raised funds for the Continental Army during the Revolutionary War and were responsible, in part, for financing the development of the District of Columbia and early American universities such as Harvard, Yale, Columbia, and Dartmouth.[4]

Yet, despite some of the developments made possible by the revenues generated through lotteries, many colonists had strong moral objections to gambling. For example, the Puritans, who settled much of New England, opposed gambling because they believed it undermined the "Protestant ethic" of self-control, hard work, and thrift. Many religious leaders of the time also condemned gambling because they believed it destroyed families and communities, and exposed gamblers to other vices such as alcohol and prostitution.[5]

Eventually, most forms of gambling and all lotteries were outlawed by the states beginning in the 1870s following tremendous scandals in the Louisiana lottery. However, in an effort to invigorate a lagging economy, the state of Nevada once again legalized casino gambling in 1931, while the revival of lotteries began in 1964 when New Hampshire established a state lottery.[6] Currently, all states, with the exception of Hawaii and Utah, offer some type of legalized gambling.

Overall, gambling in the United States has transitioned from early acceptance to prohibition to widespread proliferation. Viewed as a legitimate, socially acceptable form of entertainment, today legalized gambling generates more revenues than any other popular leisure-time activity.[7] Statistics indicate that approximately 85 percent of all Americans have gambled at least once in their lives and between 65–80 percent reported having gambled in the past year.[8]

For most individuals, gambling is a relaxing activity that does not result in negative consequences. Unfortunately, however, for some individuals gambling becomes more than harmless fun. The most severe form of gambling, pathological gambling, is recognized as a mental health condition. The personal and social effects of pathological gambling often include significant financial losses, family problems, legal and employment difficulties, psychological distress, and suicide.[9]

While the consequences of pathological gambling are certainly disturbing, there also exists an equally unsettling trend with respect to the growth in the population of pathological gamblers. Statistics indicate that the prevalence of the disorder is on the rise. In 1976, it was estimated that the base rate of the US adult population that constituted pathological gamblers was 0.77;[10] however, today studies estimate that approximately 5–6 percent of the adult gambling population experiences significant problems as a result of gambling.[11]

Definitions

Often referred to as gaming, gambling can be defined as placing something of value at risk in the hopes of gaining something of greater value. Gambling is a behavior that occurs on a continuum ranging from no involvement to excessive involvement. Locations along the behavioral continuum have been demarcated using terms such as at-risk, subclinical, problem, pathological, compulsive, and in-transition.[12]

Individuals experiencing difficulties with gambling can generally be grouped into two categories: *problem gamblers* and *pathological* or *compulsive gamblers*. Despite some distinctions, the terms are often used interchangeably in the gambling literature. All three designations are used to describe a disorder that is characterized by loss of control over gambling, deception regarding the extent of one's involvement with gambling, family and job disruption, theft, and "chasing" losses or attempting to win back money that has been lost while gambling.[13]

The term *pathological* generally refers to those individuals whose gambling behavior meets at least five of the ten diagnostic criteria outlined in the American Psychiatric Association's (APA) *Diagnostic Statistical Manual of Mental Disorders, Fourth Edition-Text Revision*. The term *problem gambling* is generally reserved for those individuals whose behavior meets three of the *DMS-IV-TR* diagnostic criteria. The term *compulsive gambling* is most frequently used by laypersons such as members of Gamblers Anonymous (GA); however, the term *compulsive gambling* does meet the *pathological gambling* diagnostic criteria. Additionally, the term *disordered gambling* is also often used in the literature to identify problem and/or pathological gambling behavior. A meta-analysis of studies encompassing the years 1975–1999 revealed that 1.9 percent of North American adults qualified for a lifetime diagnosis of pathological gambling, while 4.2 percent fell into the problem gambler category.[14]

Classification

Although first mentioned in the medical literature in the early 1800s, the APA did not classify pathological gambling as a psychiatric disorder until 1980 when it debuted in the *DSM-III*. Along with pyromania, kleptomania, trichotillomania, and intermittent explosive disorder, pathological gambling is currently classified as an impulse control disorder not elsewhere specified. The diagnostic criteria include ten items.

The Hidden Addiction

Many of the current diagnostic criteria for pathological gambling share features with those of substance use disorders. For example, tolerance, withdrawal, repeated unsuccessful attempts to cut back or quit, and interference in major areas of life function are diagnostic criteria associated with both pathological gambling and substance use disorders. These similarities have led some clinicians and scholars to both challenge pathological gambling's present classification in the *DSM-IV-TR* as an impulse control disorder and, instead, argue for its reclassification as an addiction in the forthcoming *DSM-5*.[15]

The term *addiction* is usually used to explain a compulsive attraction or pathological attachment to a substance, normally a drug. However, researchers and clinicians now recognize that some individuals can become addicted to certain behaviors, such as sex, eating, and gambling. All addiction is characterized by a loss of control, preoccupation, compulsivity, narrowing of interests, dishonesty, guilt and chronic relapse. Addictions to behavioral processes are called behavioral addictions or process addictions.[16]

Pathological gambling is often referred to as the "hidden addiction" because it manifests no obvious physical signs of addictive behavior, i.e., no needle marks, slurred speech, alcohol on the breath, or dilated pupils. A urinalysis, Breathalyzer test, or blood test will not reveal a problem. Consequently, a gambling disorder is significantly more difficult to detect than a substance use disorder, a factor that makes early intervention difficult. Finding it easier to conceal their addiction, individuals often progress more easily and, often, more rapidly toward the pathological end of the gambling-behavior continuum.[17]

The Course of Pathological Gambling

The degree to which an individual gambles or wagers varies along several dimensions. If examined over time, an individual's gambling activities and problems can decrease, increase, remain at the same level, or recur.[18] Based on the results of two surveys, the Gambling Impact and Behavior Study (GIBS) and the National Epidemiologic Survey on Alcohol and Related Conditions (NESARC), Wendy Slutske concluded that the trajectory of pathological gambling is best described as "variable."[19]

Gambling behavior can occur on different levels and progress through different phases. Shafer et al. demarcated four levels ranging from zero to three in order to illustrate the various degrees of gambling involvement.[20] Custer and Milt identified three phases—the winning phase, the losing phase, and the desperation phase—in order to describe the course of progression.[21] Recently, an additional phase—the hopeless phase—was added.[22] Not all gamblers experience all levels or phases, nor is the progression though which individuals traverse necessarily linear.

Levels of Gambling[23]

- **Level 0 Gambling:** Refers to individuals who have never gambled.

- **Level 1 Gambling:** Refers to "social" or "recreational' gambling; it is gambling to a degree that does not result in any significant problems. This categorization describes the vast majority of the population.

- **Level 2 Gambling:** Refers to wagering to such an extent that some gambling-related problems have developed. This type of gambling is also referred to as at-risk gambling, in-transition gambling, and problem gambling.

- **Level 3 Gambling:** Refers to gambling to a degree that is associated with significant problems. Individuals gambling at Level 3 typically meet the *DSM-IV-TR* diagnostic criteria for pathological gambling.

Phases of Gambling[24]

- **The Winning Phase:** During this initial phase, individuals find betting fun, exciting, social, or a way to escape daily stressors of life. Occasionally, individuals win large sums of money during this phase which generally leads to betting larger amounts and spending more time gambling.

- **The Losing Phase:** In the second phase, the gambler becomes preoccupied with gambling and the need for placing larger bets more frequently. Losses increase but are rationalized as a "losing streak." During this phase, individuals begin to "chase" their losses, lie about the extent of their involvement, and experience gambling-related difficulties, as well as make and break promises to self and others to quit gambling.

- **The Desperation Phase:** During this third phase, the gambler may experience the onset of health problems and relationships may begin to deteriorate. Feelings of desperation and hopelessness ensue as losses continue to mount. He or she continues to cling to the fantasy of winning, making it more difficult to quit. The gambler may steal, write bad checks, or commit other crimes in order to finance gambling.

- **The Hopeless Phase:** In this phase, the gambler no longer believes that there is hope or help. The gambler gives up; he or she does not care if he or she lives or dies. Jail or prison becomes a possibility. Depression is common, and suicide is a real risk.

Action and Escape Gamblers

Custer delineated the compulsive gambler characterization into two sub-type categories.[25] Often, a compulsive gambler will fit neatly into one of two general categories: *action gamblers* and *escape gamblers*. More often, however, an individual will present with characteristics that represent a combination of one of the following two categories:[26]

- **Action gambler:** An action gambler generally prefers games that require some skill. Highly competitive, this individual usually has a background in sports. Gambling is an activity endeavored in order to beat another individual or the house; consequently, the action gambler thinks that it is possible to develop a system in order to achieve this goal. For an action gambler, gambling activities generally begin in adolescence and continue into adulthood. Games of choice may include poker, blackjack, craps or other dice games, horse racing, stock market trading, or sports betting.

- **Escape gambler:** An escape gambler typically chooses games that do not require high levels of skill or knowledge. Rather, games of "luck," e.g., slot machines, video poker, bingo, etc., are preferred. Gambling behavior generally begins as a form of recreation, a means of socialization, or as a method of distraction in order to escape from problems. While gambling, the escape gambler may enter a trancelike state and spend excessive amounts of time "lost" in gambling.

Etiology

Over time, several models have been constructed in order to explain or describe the development of gambling disorders. Early models included learning, cognitive, genetic, and emotion-based theories.[27] Although these models certainly provided insight and a deeper understanding of each of these variables related to the development of problem gambling, they had limited descriptive, explanative, and predictive value. Due to their one-dimensional nature, they were unable to fully account for all of the complexities related to the development of pathological gambling.

Today, pathological gambling is understood as a complex, multifaceted, and multidimensional phenomenon. It is generally considered a heterogeneous disorder in which multiple variables interact in multiple manners. Evidence now exists that biological, psychological, and social factors are all relevant to the development of problematic levels of gambling.[28]

To date, no one single theory has been developed to explain the onset and maintenance of disordered gambling or account for all the permutations of problem gambling behavior.[29] However, several, more comprehensive models have been developed in recent years. Unlike earlier theories, these models seek to both identify the multiple etiological factors involved in the development of pathological gambling, as well as describe the relationships between these variables.

General Theory of Addictions

The General Theory of Addictions, developed by Jacobs in 1986, was the first to attempt to account for both physiological and psychological factors in the etiology of pathological gambling and other addictive behaviors.[30] The model suggests that excessive substance use and/or excessive behaviors, such as gambling, represent maladaptive coping skills.[31] The need or desire to escape from one's problems usually occurs more frequently among individuals who have poorly developed coping skills.[32]

The General Theory of Addictions proposes that pathological gamblers possess two interrelated sets of predisposing factors: 1) a physiological resting state of arousal that is either hypotensive (depressed) or hypertensive (anxious) and 2) a psychological vulnerability toward feelings of inadequacy, low self-esteem, and low self-efficacy that generally developed as a result of early rejection from caregivers and peers, which, in turn, foster a need for recognition and approval. These predisposing factors, in combination with a need for escape and wish-fulfillment, cause an individual to experiment with substances and behaviors that make him or her feel normal. In order to avoid returning to aversive affective states, an individual will continue the behavior, in this case, gambling, in such a manner that it becomes habituated and subsequently, resistant to extinction.[33]

Pathways Model

In 2002, Blaszczynski and Nower proposed the *Pathways Model*. The model maintains that the interplay of multiple factors leads to problem gambling behavior. However, unlike other theories, the model suggests that problem gamblers are not a homogenous population. Although individuals may share a number of common ecological factors, such as cognitive distortions, behavioral contingencies of reinforcement, access to gambling opportunities, etc., they differ with respect to other important biopsychosocial factors.[34] Consequently, the Pathways Model suggests that there are at least three subgroups of problem and pathological gamblers presenting with distinct etiological processes and clinical features. The three pathways are summarized as follows:[35, 36]

- **Pathway 1:** Behaviorally conditioned problem gamblers. These individuals do not necessarily demonstrate psychiatric pathology. Instead, these individuals fall prey to a highly addictive schedule of behavioral reinforcement.

- **Pathway 2:** Emotionally vulnerable problem gamblers. These individuals tend to manifest both a biological and psychological vulnerability to pathology characterized by high levels of depression and/or anxiety and a history of poor social support, low self-esteem, and a history of familial neglect or abuse.

- **Pathway 3:** Antisocial impulsivist problem gamblers. These individuals possess psychosocial and biologically based vulnerabilities similar to Pathway 2, but also manifest impulsive and antisocial tendencies.

Public Health Model

Shaffer and Korn have described a public health approach to gambling.[37] Like most public health matters, there is a complex relationship between multiple determinants in which the confluence of variables has the capacity to produce a variety of outcomes ranging from desirable to undesirable. Consequently, the public health model recognizes that gambling generates both positive and negative consequences that affect all aspects of the community, including health and socioeconomic dimensions.

Similar to the public health models used for alcohol, tobacco, and other drugs, this paradigm is not restricted to a narrow focus on addiction. Instead, it offers a broad viewpoint by describing the complex interrelationships and interactions between a number of variables that are all related to the development of pathological gambling. The specific variables relative to this model are the host, the agent, and the vector/environment.

With respect to gambling, the host is defined as the individual who decides to gamble. He or she might be at risk for developing problems based upon his or her own particular neurobiology, psychology, and behavior patterns. The agent represents the gambling activities. The vector refers to the money and the environment represents both micro levels and macro levels. The gambling venue, family, and local community in which the host resides are elements contained within the microenvironment. The components included in the macroenvironment are the socioeconomic, cultural, social policy, and political context within which the gambling occurs, i.e., whether gambling is legal or not, the degree of accessibility or availability, and whether or not it is socially sanctioned or promoted.

Neurobiology

Although neurobiological studies related to pathological gambling are still in their infancy, preliminary results indicate that pathological gambling and substance use disorders share neurobiological underpinnings.[38] Both psychoactive drugs (e.g., alcohol, cocaine, heroin, etc.) and behaviors (e.g., gambling) have the capacity to stimulate neurobiological systems. For example, the results from functional magnetic resonance imaging (fMRI) studies have revealed that the manner in which money and beauty energize the reward system is similar to that associated with the anticipating of cocaine among users.[39]

A growing body of literature supports the hypothesis that several neurotransmitter systems related to arousal, mood regulation, and reward regulation may all play a role with respect to impulsivity, mood disorders, and impaired control. As described in detail in the previous chapter, research results have implicated the noradrenergic, serotonergic, and dopaminergic neurotransmitter systems in the pathophysiology of behavioral addictions and substance use disorders.[40] Central noradrenaline (norepinephrine) is involved in the physiological functions associated with arousal and impulse control.[41] Serotonergic function is linked to behavioral initiation, inhibition, and aggression, while dopaminergic function is associated with reward and reinforcement mechanisms.[42]

Several brain circuits that have been implicated in the development of addictive behavior have also been studied in pathological gambling. Four have been found to be of particular interest: 1) the "reward" circuit, which is located in the nucleus accumbens; 2) the "motivational and drive" circuit, which is located in the orbitofrontal cortex; 3) the "memory and learning" circuit, which is located in the amygdala and the hippocampus; and 4) the "control" circuit, which is located in the dorsolateral prefrontal cortex and the anterior cingulated gyrus.[43] Additionally, neuropsychological studies of pathological gamblers have demonstrated that pathological gamblers have deficits in the frontal lobe reward system, leading investigators to hypothesize that impairment of executive function may play a role in the etiology of pathological gambling.[44]

Genetics

Research results now suggest that there is a likely genetic vulnerability to pathological gambling. While the specific phenotype through which such vulnerability is expressed remains unknown, genetic studies suggest that the possession of the dopamine D2A1 allele receptor gene may result in deficits in the dopamine reward pathways. This deficit may prompt affected individuals to seek pleasure-generating activities and, consequently, place them at high risk for the development of multiple addictive, impulsive, and compulsive behaviors including substance abuse, binge eating, sex addiction, and pathological gambling.[45]

Risk Factors

In addition to neurobiological and genetic vulnerabilities, several other risk factors have been identified with respect to the development of pathological gambling. Some of the risk factors associated with the development of pathological gambling include earlier age of onset, male gender, social modeling, i.e., the gambling attitudes and behaviors of parents and peers;[46] personality factors, i.e., impulsivity and sensation-seeking traits[47] and antisocial behaviors;[48] ineffective coping strategies;[49] and pre-existing mood disorders, anxiety disorders, and/or substance abuse disorders, low self-esteem, and lack of social support.[50] However, it is important to remember that, as with other addictions and behaviors, it is the interaction between a variety of factors, and not those factors alone, that may put an individual at higher risk for developing a problem with gambling. Therefore, risk factors cannot be assumed to be causative factors.

Trauma

While histories of abuse and trauma have been frequently reported by individuals diagnosed with substance use disorders, a linkage between problem gambling and trauma is appearing in the literature with increasing frequency. Gambling has been characterized as a way of coping with trauma and abuse, especially among women.[51] In a study conducted with pathological gamblers undergoing treatment, Kausch et al. found that 64.4 percent reported some history of abuse, 56.8 percent reported a history of emotional abuse, 40.5 percent reported physical abuse, and 24.3 percent reported a history of sexual abuse. Multiple abuses (two or more incidents) were reported by 42.3 percent of the gamblers, and both physical and sexual abuse histories were reported by 16.2 percent of the sample. Women were significantly more likely to report abuse than men in this sample.[52]

Erroneous Cognitions

Many studies have supported the theory that cognitive distortions or irrational beliefs may play a role in the development and maintenance of both addictive behaviors in general and pathological gambling specifically. Despite the objective, statistical probability related to games of chance, problem gamblers tend to maintain inaccurate perceptions about their ability to control or influence the gambling outcomes. Cognitive distortions associated with disordered gambling include: 1) the gambler's fallacy, i.e., the belief that completely random events, such as the outcome of a coin toss, are influenced by recent events;[53] 2) illusions of control, i.e., superstitious behaviors by which the gambler thinks that he or she has a reliable means of manipulating the event outcome in his or her favor;[54] 3) the magnification of gambling skills, i.e., exaggerated self-confidence;[55] and 4) recall bias, i.e., the tendency to remember and overestimate wins while forgetting about, underestimating, or rationalizing losses.[56]

Accessibility

The relationship between accessibility to gambling settings and gambling problems is controversial. A study conducted by Gerstein et al.[57] found that the prevalence rates of both problem and pathological gambling was double that of the general population for individuals living within fifty miles of a casino. However, it is not possible to determine precisely what role, if any, location plays in the development of disordered gambling. While it is possible that the availability of or access to gambling opportunities may increase an individual's vulnerability for developing a gambling problem, it is also possible that individuals with a gambling problem may relocate to areas that feature multiple gambling opportunities. Furthermore, it is equally possible that casinos locate in areas where the population has already demonstrated high rates of disordered gambling.[58]

Comorbidity

Comorbidity is the term used to describe the co-occurrence of two or more disorders. Each disorder can occur independently, a pattern identified as *lifetime comorbidity*, or two disorders can occur simultaneously, a pattern known as *current comorbidity*.[59] There is a high incidence of associated comorbid disorders and pathological gambling. Comorbid disorders for pathological gambling include substance use disorders, attention-deficit hyperactivity disorder (ADHD), antisocial, narcissistic, and borderline personality disorders, depression, cyclothymia, and bipolar disorder.[60] In addition, pathological gamblers frequently engage in multiple impulsive and dysfunctional behaviors such as compulsive shopping and compulsive sexual behavior.[61] Suicide is also highly associated with gambling disorders.[62]

Substance Abuse

Research has shown that individuals using alcohol and/or other drugs are six times more likely than the general population to either experience a gambling problem or to develop a gambling problem as a result of what Blume termed "switching addictions,"[63] meaning that an individual will cease one addiction or behavior but, subsequently, in the process, develop a different one. The rate of probable pathological gamblers among substance abusers ranges from 10–33 percent; 47 percent of inpatient pathological gamblers have been shown to be substance abusers. Fifty-two percent of GA members have been shown to be alcohol and/or other drug abusers.[64] Cigarette smoking is also common among treatment-seeking gamblers. Studies indicate that 37–59 percent meet diagnostic criteria for nicotine dependence.[65] According to the results of a recent study, the onset of a substance use disorder preceded the onset of a gambling disorder for the majority of gamblers presenting with comorbid disorders.

Affective disorders

Pathological gambling is highly comorbid with affective disorders. Among inpatient samples of pathological gambling patients, 76 percent met criteria for a major depressive disorder, 38 percent were hypomanic, 8 percent were manic, and 2 percent were diagnosed with schizoaffective disorder of the depressive type. In outpatient samples, 28 percent of pathological gambling patients met the criteria for major depressive disorder, 24 percent for bipolar disorder, and 28 percent for anxiety disorder.[66]

ADHD

Pathological gambling has been associated with ADHD. Twenty percent of pathological gamblers have comorbid ADHD. Additionally, there is an increased frequency of childhood onset AD/HD.[67]

With respect to comorbidity, it is necessary to remember that the statistics represent correlations. Determining a causal role, if any exists, is difficult, if not impossible. For instance, do substance abusers gamble or do gamblers abuse substances? Do individuals with a psychological disorder(s) gamble to self-medicate their emotional discord or does the stress generated by gambling-related problems facilitate the development of psychological disorders?[68] Regardless of the order of onset, however, it is possible that all three—substance abuse disorders, psychological disorders, and gambling disorders—may interact and subsequently perpetuate one another.[69]

Crime

Research has established a link between crime and gambling behavior.[70] In the US, a 1996 study by Thompson, Gazel, and Rickman found that, on average, the serious problem gambler lost nearly $100,000 and owed $38,644 before seeking help. As finances diminish, gamblers may resort to crime in order to pay debts, maintain appearances, and acquire more money with which to gamble. It is estimated that 21–85 percent of pathological gamblers commit crimes such as fraud, theft, embezzlement, forgery, robbery, assault, and blackmail.[71] During the 1980s and 1990s, studies reported that between 12.5–15 percent of all pathological gamblers would become incarcerated.[72] However, as with comorbidity, it is difficult to separate cause from effect. In other words, do criminals gamble or do gamblers become criminals?[73]

Bankruptcy

A high percentage of gamblers will also face bankruptcy. According to the Gambling Impact Behavior Study (GIBS) conducted in 1998, nearly 25 percent of both problem and pathological gamblers filed for bankruptcy compared to 5.5 percent of social gamblers and 4.2 percent of nongamblers. Additionally, pathological gamblers in that study reported rates of indebtedness that were 25 percent greater than those of social gamblers and 120 percent greater than nongamblers.[74]

Suicide

The negative consequences and losses associated with gambling problems may act as catalysts for suicidal ideation and behaviors. Under the intense pressure of both emotional distress and financial stress, some individuals may view suicide as the only viable solution to their problem(s). Although a causal link has not been established, there is emerging evidence that gambling severity increases the risk of both suicidal ideation and behavior. Lesieur and Klein suggested that pathological gamblers were five to ten times more likely to attempt suicide than the general population. Studies involving treatment-seeking pathological gamblers found that 36–50 percent had a history of suicidal ideation,[75, 76] and 20–30 percent of pathological gamblers have made suicide attempts.[77] Moreover, the mood and substance use disorders that commonly co-occur with pathological gambling are also highly associated with suicide,[78] thereby further increasing an individual's vulnerability for suicidal ideation and/or attempts.

However, the role that gambling itself plays in precipitating suicidal ideation and/or behaviors remains unclear. Studies have generated mixed and inconclusive results. For example, while Otto Kausch, a forensic psychiatrist, found that 64.3 percent of the study's suicide attempters reported that their most recent suicide attempt was related to gambling, a study by Hodgins et al.[79] revealed that suicide attempts were nearly universally made when participants reported feeling depressed and, more than half the time, were made under the influence of alcohol or other drugs. Furthermore, ideation tended to predate the onset of gambling problems by ten years in this sample. Based on these contradictory findings, it appears that gambling problems are but one of a number of stressors that may contribute to suicidal ideation and attempts.[80]

Special Populations

Historically, pathological gambling has been viewed as a male-dominated problem. Today, however, it is clear that individuals experiencing gambling problems are not comprised of a homogeneous group. Rather, excessive gambling affects individuals with diverse biopsychosocial profiles and cuts across age, gender, ethnicity, and social class.

Gender

Studies indicate that women make up the fastest growing group seeking help for problem gambling.[81] An estimated one-third of problem gamblers are now women.[82] Although the age of onset for problem gambling in women generally occurs later than in men, women are found to experience a more rapid progression into a gambling problem than men, a phenomenon referred to as *telescoping*.[83] While women tend to initiate gambling activities at a later age than men, women tend to seek treatment for problem gambling earlier than men.[84]

A number of researchers have reported both type and motivational gambling-related gender differences between male and female gamblers. In general, males are more likely to play games that require "skill," e.g., card games, horse race betting, and sports betting, while females are more likely to play games of "luck," e.g., slot and video poker machines, bingo, keno, etc.[85] While men tend to be intrigued by the "action" associated with gambling, women tend to use gambling as an "escape" mechanism. Commonly, female pathological gamblers cite escape from personal pressures, boredom, and depression as reasons for gambling.[86]

Adolescents

Gambling by teenagers is not a new phenomenon; however, according to one study, adolescents of the 1990s were the first US generation reared in a culture in which gambling was believed to be not only an acceptable activity, but a career option as well.[87] As a result of society's more permissive attitude toward gambling, adolescent gambling prevalence rates are on the rise.

During the 1980s, it was estimated that 45 percent of adolescents had gambled during the previous year.[88] Today, multiple surveys of middle and high school age students in North America now suggest that between 60–80 percent have engaged in some form of gambling for money over the past year. Furthermore, it is estimated that of those who gamble, 10–15 percent are at risk for developing a gambling problem.[89] These rates are significantly higher than those reported in the general adult population. In fact, research results indicate that adolescents experience this problem at approximately 2.5 to 3 times the rate of their adult counterparts.[90]

Seniors

Older adults comprise one of the fastest growing segments of the population. Consequently, this particular demographic represents an attractive target for gaming operators. In fact, over the past several decades, the growth rate of gambling participation has been highest among the older adult age group, increasing from 35 percent in 1975 to 80 percent in 1998.[91]

Seniors may be especially vulnerable to developing a gambling problem for a number of reasons. First, seniors tend to have much more discretionary time available than individuals within the general population. Second, the desire to numb or escape from the uncomfortable feelings associated with life changes, e.g., death of a spouse, health or financial problems, loneliness, boredom, or depression, may motivate some seniors to gamble. Third, seniors may be at higher risk of developing a gambling problem by virtue of greater accessibility to gambling opportunities than the general population. Bus trips or group excursions organized and/or sponsored by senior living centers are popular activities among this population. Fourth, many seniors live on a fixed income. Consequently, financial losses can have greater impact. As a result, financial stresses can escalate more quickly, which in turn, may make seniors more vulnerable to maintaining or increasing their gambling activities in order to "chase" their losses.[92]

Assessment

A variety of instruments have been developed for screening and classifying gambling behaviors. The most widely used instrument for the general screening of gambling disorders is the South Oaks Gambling Screen.[93] The SOGS is highly correlated to the *DSM-IV-TR* diagnosis of pathological gambling. The instrument consists of twenty items that assess the presence of gambling problems. Scores range from zero to twenty. A score of three or more indicates that the client is a "potential pathological gambler," and a score of five or more is indicative of a "probable pathological gambler."[94] Although demonstrated to be valid and reliable, the SOGS has been criticized for its tendency to generate false positives. In other words, the SOGS may overstate the number of pathological gamblers.[95]

The opposite is true of the NODS, National Opinion Research Center DSM Screen for Gambling Problems. In other words, NODS tends to generate false negatives; consequently, it tends to underestimate the number of pathological gamblers.[96] The NODS defines ten problem areas based on the ten diagnostic criteria for pathological gambling listed in the *DSM-IV-TR*.[97] Originally developed as a survey instrument for research purposes, it is suggested that clinicians supplement any information from NODS with a full clinical interview.[98]

Because of its brevity, the two-question Lie/Bet Questionnaire has also been used to screen for gambling problems. A positive response to either or both questions generally indicates a gambling problem. The questions are as follows: 1) "Have you ever had to lie to people important to you about how much you gambled?" and 2) "Have you ever felt the need to bet more and more money?"

However, one of the best known measures of compulsive gambling is not a traditional psychometric inventory but, rather, the Gamblers Anonymous twenty questions. According to GA, most compulsive gamblers answer yes to at least seven of the twenty questions. While it is a viable screening tool, like the SOGS and other self-report inventories, individuals can easily misrepresent themselves when responding.[99]

Treatment

Despite its increasing prevalence, pathological gambling often remains untreated. While effective treatment for gambling problems does exist, relatively few individuals experiencing gambling problems seek treatment.[100] Analysis of data from two large national surveys conducted in the US indicated that approximately only 7–10 percent of lifetime pathological gamblers had sought treatment or attended GA.[101] Conversely, this means that between 90–93 percent of the individuals experiencing gambling problems do not seek treatment.

Although an individual may recognize that he or she has developed a problem with gambling, there are internal and external barriers to seeking help. Suuvali et al. conducted a literature review in order to identify the obstacles that prevent problem gamblers from seeking treatment for their gambling problem. The results of the study indicated that the most commonly reported barriers to seeking treatment were as follows: 1) a desire to handle the problem by oneself; 2) shame/embarrassment/stigma; 3) a reluctance to admit to the problem; and, 4) practical issues related to attending treatment, i.e., time and money concerns.[102]

The reasons for ceasing addictive behaviors, and subsequently seeking treatment, can be attributed to both internal and external categories. Internal motivations are generally more predictive of long-term success than are external motivations. In a 2002 study conducted by Hodgins et al., the predominant internal reasons for quitting gambling included emotional factors, concerns about family/children, financial reasons, fear of future negative consequences, and the experience of hitting "rock bottom." External motivators included legal and work-related problems. Suurvali et al. found that help-seeking occurred largely in response to either impending or existing gambling-related harms, i.e., financial problems, relationship issues, and negative emotions.[103]

Lipinski et al. examined the reviews of psychological treatments for pathological gambling and generated three conclusions. First, pathological gambling responds to psychosocial treatment. Interventions falling within the cognitive-behavioral spectrum have the most empirical support at present.[104] Second, brief outpatient treatments have been successful with other addictive behaviors and show promise for the treatment of pathological gambling. Third, positive change from psychological treatment is not limited to abstinence-only outcomes; rather, the reduction of gambling behaviors to a more normal or functional level has been demonstrated to be a viable treatment goal option for some.[105]

Both process addictions and substance use disorders often respond favorably to the same treatments. The cognitive-behavioral therapy (CBT), motivational enhancement, and twelve-step approaches commonly used to treat substance use disorders have been used successfully to treat pathological gambling. The psychosocial interventions for both behavioral addictions and substance use disorders often rely on a relapse prevention model that encourages abstinence by identifying patterns of abuse, avoiding or coping with high-risk situations, and making lifestyle changes that reinforce healthier behaviors.[106]

Cognitive behavioral treatments generally take one of two approaches. The first approach works toward the goal of total abstinence. The second approach works from a perspective known as harm reduction, the goal of which is to learn how to modify and/or control gambling behavior.[107]

The basic tenets of CBT suggest that a relationship exists between cognitive, behavioral, and emotional factors in human functioning. Cognitive therapy perceives psychological problems as stemming from commonplace processes such as faulty thinking, making incorrect inferences on the basis of inadequate or incorrect information, and failing to distinguish between fantasy and reality.[108] The central assumption underlying the cognitive-behavioral approach for pathological gambling is that pathological gamblers will continue to gamble in spite of repeated losses given that they maintain an unrealistic belief that losses can be recovered. This perspective assumes that a number of erroneous beliefs (e.g., illusions of control, the gambler's fallacy, failure to understand chance, and the independence of events) foster persistent gambling behavior.[109]

Cognitive behavioral therapy is designed to identify and modify both erroneous cognitions, as well as to identify and modify poor coping responses.[110] Therefore, CBT for disordered gambling aims to help problem gamblers understand all the facets of their problem in order to remedy it. The therapy uses an educational approach intended to enhance coping skills directly by teaching skills, rehearsing with role plays in-session, and practicing newly developed skills between sessions using homework exercises.[111] The CBT model most frequently used for impulse control disorders consists of four components: 1) cognitive restructuring to correct irrational and dysfunctional beliefs that precede impulsive behavior; 2) the acquisition/development of problem-solving skills aimed at generating alternative responses to stress; 3) social skills training; and 4) relapse prevention in which the client is taught to identify, avoid, and/or cope with high-risk situations.[112] The treatment not only helps individuals to meet their goal, i.e., abstinence or controlled gambling, but it also helps clients to cope with the many consequences related to excessive gambling. As a result, individuals acquire or develop the skills and attitudes that they can apply in daily life.[113]

Motivational interviewing (MI), developed by Miller and later elaborated on by Miller and Rollnick, has also been used in treating pathological gambling. Motivational interviewing uses both directive and client-centered counseling styles that are designed to enhance the client's motivation to initiate the process of change. It blends principles drawn from motivational psychology, client-centered therapy, and the process of change that naturally occurs in recovery from addiction.[114]

With MI, client motivation is viewed as a fluid state that ebbs and flows during treatment. Ambivalence is considered to be a normal state of mind when initiating change. The goal of MI is to identify and mobilize the client's intrinsic values and goals in order to stimulate a behavior change. Direct persuasion, aggressive confrontation, and argumentation are the conceptual opposites of MI. In fact, these tactics generally increase client resistance and diminish the probability of change.[115] Rather, a therapist using MI partners with the client through the principles of empathic listening, rolling with resistance, heightening the awareness of the discrepancies between behavior and goals, and supporting the development of self-efficacy and optimism. This treatment process works to increase the client's motivation to change and encourages the use of individual strengths and resources to help solve problems.[116]

On a related note, Ladouceur et al. cautions clinicians to avoid the words "dependent," "compulsive," or "excessive" when treating problem gamblers.[117] The client must not feel like a sick person who must be treated. Instead, it is important to the recovery process for individuals to see themselves as autonomous and efficacious agents capable of both identifying or developing solutions and applying these solutions in order to take control of their behavior and change their lives.

Behavioral interventions have also been found to be useful for some individuals engaged in the recovery process. Both self-exclusion and funds-management strategies can help facilitate abstinence and/or gambling-behavior modification. For example, some casinos offer a program that allows gamblers to ban themselves from the establishment, thereby limiting an individual's access to a high-risk situation. Also, individuals can choose to limit their access to funds. Canceling credit cards, removing ATM cards and/or credit cards from their wallets, limiting the amount of cash carried on their person, and utilizing direct-deposit for their paychecks are all useful strategies that can be employed during the recovery process.[118]

Although pathological gambling has its own unique elements, it also manifests many signs and symptoms consistent with other disorders. Additionally, as noted above, comorbidity with other disorders is high. From this perspective, Korn and Shafer suggest that the most effective treatments for gambling problems will reflect a multimodal "cocktail approach" combined with client-treatment matching. These multidimensional treatments should include combinations of psychopharmacology, psychotherapy, and financial, educational, and self-help interventions. The variety of treatment elements is both additive and interactive, and well-suited to address the multifaceted nature of gambling disorders.

As with most therapies, each intervention has its own particular set of strengths and weaknesses. No one theory or intervention can claim perfect utility or success in all cases. Additionally, it should be noted, that formal treatment is not always a necessary prerequisite for recovery, even among gamblers with severe problems.[119] Utilizing data from previous studies, Slutske found that approximately one-third of the lifetime pathological gamblers participating in the studies had recovered naturally, that is, without formal treatment.[120]

Pharmacotherapy

The evidence for the efficacy of pharmacotherapy for gambling addicts is somewhat in its infancy and, most often, research results are contradictory. Currently, there are no US Food and Drug Administration (FDA) approved medications for the treatment of pathological gambling. However, neurobiological similarities between pathological gambling and drug addiction suggest that medications used for the treatment of drug addiction might be useful in the treatment of pathological gambling.[121] For example, Naltrexone, a μ-opioid receptor (MOR) antagonist approved by the FDA for the treatment of alcoholism and opioid dependence, has shown efficacy in controlled clinical trials for the treatment of pathological gambling. Medications that alter glutamatergic activity have also been used to treat both behavioral addictions and substance use disorders.[122] Selective serotonin reuptake inhibitors (SSRIs) have also shown some promise with respect to reducing the craving to gamble.[123]

Gamblers Anonymous (GA)

A less formal, but commonly utilized intervention for problem gambling is the mutual-aid fellowship called Gamblers Anonymous. Founded in Los Angeles, California in 1957 and modeled on the Twelve-Steps of the Alcoholics Anonymous (AA) program, GA is a self-help group for compulsive gamblers[124] that contains cognitive and spiritual components that facilitate the recovery process.

Although GA is a popular intervention for pathological gambling, high rates of attrition limit its efficacy. Most research demonstrates that the vast majority of GA attendees fail to become actively involved in the fellowship. A study conducted in 1988 by Stewart and Brown found that only 18 percent of the sample attended GA meetings regularly for a year or more. Of all the new members in the study, only 7.5 percent attained a one-year abstinence pin, and 7.3 percent received a two-year pin.[125]

According to GA, success is characterized as complete abstinence from gambling for a period of at least two years. However, some data suggest that the effectiveness of GA can be enhanced by participation in professional treatment programs. Research results indicate that attendance at GA, coupled with engagement in professional therapy, was associated with long-term abstinence.[126]

Relapse

Similar to addiction to alcohol and other drugs, pathological gambling is characterized as a chronic relapsing disorder. Relapse rates, in general, range from 80–90 percent in the first year following treatment.[127] Relapse does not occur without a reason. There are many contributing factors, as well as warning signs, that indicate an individual may be in danger of relapsing. In an analysis of relapse episodes obtained from clients with a variety of addictive behavior problems, Marlatt and Gordon identified three high-risk situations that were associated with almost 75 percent of the relapses reported: negative emotional states, interpersonal conflict, and social pressure.

The disruptive effects of relapse are profound; therefore, relapse prevention should be integrated into therapy and addressed throughout the entire therapeutic process. Relapse prevention strategies should focus on the following two objectives: 1) help individuals prevent relapse, and 2) help individuals manage a relapse should one occur. Frequently experienced as traumatic events, relapses are generally accompanied by intense feelings of guilt and shame. Therefore, if a relapse occurs, rather than view it as a catastrophe or failure, clients should be encouraged to use it to their advantage by consolidating their gains and identifying the precipitants that led them to choose to gamble again.

Prevention

Problematic gambling results in far-reaching and long-lasting negative consequences; therefore, prevention is a primary factor when addressing the issue. While prevention efforts are critical in protecting youth, adults, and seniors from developing serious problems, the specific type of prevention approach or approaches that should be adopted remains unclear. The central questions currently being asked pertain to which form of prevention is best for targeting the issue of gambling problems.[128]

There are two global paradigms under which particular prevention approaches can be classified: *abstinence* or *harm reduction*. While these two approaches are not mutually exclusive, they are predicated upon different short-term goals and processes. Essentially, the strategies employed by harm reduction policies, programs, and interventions seek to assist individuals experiencing gambling-related difficulties without demanding abstinence. The primary objective of most programs is to foster awareness of gambling in general, as well as to provide information about problem gambling, its warning signs, consequences associated with excessive gambling, and how or where to get help for an individual who has developed a gambling problem. Most governments today have implemented a harm reduction approach aimed at reducing or minimizing the negative impact of gambling without negating gaming revenues or access to the general public.[129]

Conclusion

Gambling is embedded in a cultural and social context, as well as in a psychological one. Although most gambling research has focused on its adverse mental health and social consequences, gambling does generate positive benefits for both individuals and society as a whole. For example, gambling can, for some, provide an opportunity to socialize, engender a sense of connectedness, or offer a respite from life's daily demands. Health benefits can also accrue to communities through gambling-related economic development. For instance, casinos can be a catalyst for economic development.[130]

Most individuals who gamble are able to do so socially or recreationally without generating negative consequences. However, a small percentage of the gambling population does develop serious problems with gambling and, as a result, experiences significant consequences. Excessive gambling has the potential to disrupt an individual's function in all spheres of life. Pathological gambling is associated with increased physical and psychological distress, psychiatric comorbidity, financial and legal difficulties, academic and/or employment disruptions, and familial and/or relational discord.

Much of the research into pathological gambling is preliminary. However, data indicate that, like substance use disorders, disordered gambling is amenable to treatment. However, research efforts need to be expanded considerably in order to further develop and improve both prevention and treatment efforts.

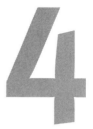

Sexual Addiction

Larry Ashley, EdS, LCADC, CPGC

Natalie Kaufman

Gina Luera

The term "sexual addiction" has been frequently misused in the media and the counseling field by attributing it to people with high sex drives and/or a history of adultery. It has been stigmatized with certain myths, lack of understanding, and acceptance in which its importance is understated as a true manifestation of addiction. There has been misunderstanding regarding the prevalence with which females become sexual addicts. It is said they can only become "love addicts" and act out from neediness. Treatment and diagnosis for sexual addiction, as well as the consequences, are the same for men and women and is another misunderstanding that stigmatizes sexual addiction.[1]

There are differing opinions from professionals whether negative sexual behavior can be classified as an addiction. According to professionals such as Lee and Kent and contributors to the *DSM-IV-TR*, sex has not been considered as a manifestation of addiction from the standpoint that it is an experience rather than a substance. It is essential to understand that the prevalence of sex addiction is approximately 3 to 6 percent in the United States.[2] A discussion and exploration on etiology, assessment, criteria, diagnosis, theories, and treatment explains that compulsive sexual behavior is an addiction. By categorizing it as such, the sex addict is less likely to be stigmatized and treatment is possible.

Definition of Sexual Addiction

Sexual addiction is described as "an intimacy disorder manifested as a compulsive cycle of preoccupation, ritualization, sexual behavior or sexual anorexia (excessive control over sexual behavior), and despair."[3] Repetitive increased/decreased sexual behaviors are used to escape and soothe feelings of significant shame, stress, pain, or trauma in a person's life. "Sex addicts will sexualize feelings and experiences that are not meant to be sexual and often lack sexual boundaries."[4] Generally, sexual addiction stems from similar framework as most addictions in regards to etiology, characteristics, and elements of the disease. The difference between alcohol and other drug addiction compared to sexual addiction (much like gambling addiction and eating disorders) is the lack of involvement of external chemicals. However, much like all addictions the brain produces similar hormones and neurotransmitters that trigger the brain's reward system and cause the sense of relief or being "high." The beginning of this disruptive cycle is created once thoughts and acts (or deprivation from sexual acts) of a sexual nature trigger the reward system and alleviate negative thoughts or feelings.

Characteristics

There are specific characteristics of the sex addict that are often present. Due to the highly secretive nature and preoccupation of this disorder, addicts will suffer socially by distancing themselves from family, friends, and loved ones in order to continue their double life. Dishonesty, lying, and infidelity cause a loss of relationships. Emotionally, sex addicts will suffer from the anxiety and stress of hiding their addiction to keep from "being found out." There is a high level of shame and guilt resulting from their sexual behaviors and also from prior pain or trauma experienced.

Defense mechanisms against shame include: rage (transfer shame onto others to keep them at a distance); contempt (blame others so the addict will not feel his or her own shame); power-seeking behavior (narcissistic behavior to gain false sense of control and self-worth due to low self-esteem and cognitive distortions); perfection-seeking behavior (giving an appearance of perfection to hide the addict's shame and addiction); transferring blame (blaming loved ones for the addict's pain and indiscretions), and internal withdrawal (dissociation, avoiding others). These defenses can be identified upon assessment and are noticeable during relapse. Extreme mood changes (highs and lows, shifting from euphoria to shame and guilt, from anxiety to dissociation) are present and correspond to the addict's position in the addiction cycle. In response to the negative coping behavior, a constant internal struggle is also manifested regarding personal values, belief systems, and spirituality.

Types of Sexual Addiction

Dr. Patrick Carnes identifies ten types of behavior for sexual addiction.[5] These behaviors are external and are acted out by the sex addict with or without a partner(s). Others can be more obsession-oriented, involving thoughts instead of actions by the sex addict. To a sex addict, these behaviors are rarely considered expressions of love and commitment; rather, they are expressions of release, power, and control. Some types of sexual behaviors (which are explained later regarding levels of sexual addiction), such as masturbation, are victimless behaviors in that they do not involve another party. Other sexual behaviors are forms of victimization, such as exhibitionism, exploitive sex, and rape because they involve others and are more intrusive and at times illegal. These ten types of behavior for sexual addiction are as follows:

- Fantasy sex is an obsessive type of sex addiction. Fantasy sex involves obsessive, intrusive, and disruptive thoughts on specific sexual fantasies. Fantasy sex creates impossible standards for a sex addict when building committed relationships that, unlike fantasies, are not perfect.

- In seductive roles sex, the addict uses the tools of manipulation and flirtation to coerce others into sex. This type of sex is not about a loving connection but succeeding in the challenge of manipulation, giving the sex addict the sense of power and control.

- Anonymous sex is when the sex addict engages in sex with strangers. Unknown factors elicit a sense of arousal in the sex addict. The goal of this type of sex is to keep the sex impersonal.

- When paying for sex, the sex addict treats sex as a purchase. Paying for sex includes phone sex, purchasing prostitution, or selling oneself as a prostitute.

- Trading sex is a method used by the sex addict as a means of working to pay a debt, such as having sex for drugs.

- Voyeuristic sex is when the sex addict becomes the observer of sexual acts via pornography from books, magazines, pictures, Internet, peep shows, or others who are unaware they are being watched having sex. Voyeurism usually will include forms of masturbation.

- Exhibitionistic sex includes flashing mostly in public, involvement in pornography or sex in public. The euphoria stems not from the act of sex, but the excitement of getting caught or actually being witnessed by others while in the act.

- Intrusive sex is a sexual behavior that is a definite form of victimization. It involves a sex addict who uses his or her authority (through work or some hierarchical system) in order to touch others in a sexual manner on their private areas such as their vagina, penis, breasts, buttocks, etc.

- Pain exchange, typically known as sadomasochism (S&M) involves inflicting or receiving pain. It is usually consensual and the excitement comes from the balance of power, i.e., being dominant or submissive.

- The final type of sexual addiction is exploitative sex. Exploitative sex is the forceful act of engaging another person in sex. Some types of exploitative sex are rape and molestation that are directed at adults or children who are vulnerable and unable to defend themselves.

Levels of Sexual Addiction

Carnes distinguished three levels of sexual addiction.[6] These levels measure the severity of sexual behaviors performed by the sex addict. *Level one* lists sexual behaviors that are not uncommon, considered "normal," and for nonaddicts, usually victimless. However, for sex addicts, these sexual behaviors have a way of resulting in negative consequences due to the compulsive nature of sexual addiction or if they "involve the victimization of others."[7] Level one behavior includes homosexuality, heterosexual relationships, the use of pornography, visiting strip shows, masturbation, and prostitution.

Level two sexual behaviors are all considered forms of "victimization." Level two behaviors include voyeurism, exhibitionism, indecent phone calls, and taking liberties on individuals. *Level three* behaviors are considered serious forms of victimization. These behaviors can be illegal and considered crimes. Level three sexual behaviors include child molestation, incest, rape, and physical violence.[8]

Sexual Addiction Cycle

"Three key barriers prevent addicts from breaking the compulsive cycle and establishing successful intimacy: shame, affect disregulation, and an inability to maintain adequate sexual boundaries."[9] There are four steps to the sexual addiction cycle: preoccupation, ritualization, compulsive sexual behavior, and despair. The more the cycle is repeated, the more the behaviors and rituals intensify.

Preoccupation, as previously discussed, is the continuous, progressive thoughts about sexual behaviors that inevitably cause disturbances in daily functioning. Preoccupation continues until the sexual behavior has been completed. The ritualization phase is the addicts' specific preparations or rituals that precede their participation in the negative sexual behavior. Rituals include, but are not limited to, cruising, driving by places to ultimately pick up prostitutes or others to take home for sex, searching for places to have sex, cruising places to find someone so that the addict can flash his or her genitalia, driving by strip clubs, or the act of showering, grooming, and dressing before the sexual behavior. Compulsive sexual behavior is the actual sexual act. Feelings of despair that stem from trauma, attachment disorder, or shame from cognitive distortions come before the individual engages in the sexual behavior. Feelings of guilt, shame, and depression can also arise after the sexual behavior.[10]

Co-occurring Disorders with Sexual Addiction

Research explains that when a diagnosis of sexual addiction is present, there is a good chance another disorder can be discovered in the same person. "In a sample of 932 sex addicts, 42 percent reported chemical dependency; 38 percent reported an eating disorder; 28 percent reported compulsive working; and 26 percent reported compulsive spending."[11] Co-occurring addictions can exist and interact with one another in ways that achieve the same desired effect. Co-occurring disorders most likely stem from the same etiology, and can be treated concurrently. Failure to treat both disorders can lead to failure in treatment or relapse.

Substance Abuse

"In the research of women and addiction, sex and alcohol (or drugs) was the most common addiction ritualized together, with sex and food running a close second."[12] Sexual addiction is frequently associated with alcohol or other drug disorders. Women who suffer from sex and substance addictions are more susceptible to acts of violence or rape. Sexual behaviors stimulate similar parts of the brain as alcohol and other drugs and can produce the same pleasure or anxiety reducing effects. Alcohol and other drugs can be included as part of the ritual before or after the negative sexual behavior. Alcohol and other drugs can be used to fight off anxieties before sexual behaviors or to "come down" from the euphoria or release after sexual behaviors have been committed. Alcohol and other drugs can also be supplemented when sexual behaviors are not able to become realized. When sexual deprivation or anorexia cannot be upheld, alcohol and other drugs could be used as a way to manage the act of sex.

Trauma

"Research has shown that 97 percent of sexual addicts have been emotionally abused as children, 72 percent were physically abused, and 81 percent were sexually abused."[13] Spiritual abuse in regards to feelings of shame toward sex is another form of trauma that can contribute to sexual addiction. "Many individuals engage in self-destructive behaviors in an attempt to survive, to cope with, or to avoid painful emotions associated with original trauma and persistently find themselves caught in a self-destructive cycle of repeating traumatic experiences."[14] Sexual obsessions and behaviors are used as a way to soothe or numb the underlying, unprocessed trauma. Past trauma as well as the sexual behaviors and obsessions are the source for shame and guilt that continue to feed the sexual addiction cycle. In order to release the individual from sexual addiction it is important to identify and process the traumatic incident.

Eating Disorders

Sex and eating are essential to the sustainability of one's life. Eating disorders can be seen as either substance or process addictions, depending on the researcher. There are six common eating disorders: anorexia, bulimia, binge eating, compulsive overeating, *bulimarexia*, and insulin hidden eating disorder. These can co-occur with any of the ten forms of sexual behaviors. They have many aspects of addiction criteria in common. Individuals can use food and sex simultaneously or they can, for instance, binge on food and be sexually anorexic to avoid intimacy, fill the emptiness they may feel, and/or to gain a sense of power. Food can also be used to calm anxieties when the sexual urge cannot be satiated.

Pathological Gambling

There is limited research on the comorbidity of sexual addiction and pathological gambling. Within the research that was found, information did show high rates of co-occurrence of pathological gambling and sexual addiction. Some research shows pathological gambling to be the main addiction that alternated with the behaviors of sexual addiction. In one study of the co-occurrence of sexual addiction and pathological gambling, it was hypothesized that "gambling was used by some subjects to numb the guilt or shame of sexual addiction or that sexual addiction disinhibited some subjects to act on the urge to gamble."[15] There was no research explaining exactly how one addiction contributed to the other. There is a need for more research on the relationship between pathological gambling and sexual addiction and its treatment.

How They Work

Co-occurring addictions can affect each other in different ways that are important to understand during diagnosis, treatment planning, and relapse prevention. "Some addiction behaviors will increase simultaneously, such as drinking and gambling, or switching one for the other at the same rate of severity." This is referred to as *cross tolerance*: when one addiction is used to "moderate, relieve, or avoid withdrawal from another addiction."[16] For instance, when recovering addicts replace alcohol with caffeine and nicotine, this is referred to as "withdrawal mediation." Replacement of one addiction with another is not uncommon. This is especially true when an addict completes treatment for one addiction, for instance, to drugs, then engages in a different form of addiction, such as sex or gambling. "Alternating addiction cycles" are when addictions stem from the same etiology, give the same effect, and are used interchangeably in phases.

Addicts can use one "less shameful" form of addiction to mask another. "Intensification" takes place when co-occurring addiction behaviors are displayed at the same time (such as using alcohol and having sex) in order to get the desired effect. Ritualizing is present when one addiction precedes the behavior of the second addiction in the ritual process (the actions before the sexual behavior is acted on). "Numbing," much like with alcohol or other drugs can be used before or after the sexual behavior to calm anxiety or come down from the sexual act. Alcohol and other drugs can also be used for disinhibition as a means to follow through on sexual acts such as prostitution. "Combining" is used to "preserve a specific high by prolonging the feeling until body gives out, then rest, recover, and repeat."[17]

Etiology

There are several theories as to the etiology of sexual addiction.

Biological

Engaging in sex addiction serves a biological purpose. When the sex addict engages in sexual behaviors, neurotransmitters are released, providing temporary reward and/or pain relief that provides an illusion of control.[18] Oxytocin is a neurohormone that plays a role in attachment, human sexual response, and obsessive-compulsive behaviors.[19] It is possible that oxytocin levels in sex addicts may be deficient or in abundance causing dysfunctional behavior.

Traumatic experiences affect the biology of the brain. When an individual experiences a traumatic experience, it increases thirst, hunger, and sexual desire, which are considered survival drives. As survival drives are increased, the dopamine levels increase in the nucleus accumbens, thus enabling the "craving" feeling in sex addicts. As the activity in the brain increases, compulsions increase.[20] When considering the etiology of an individual's sex addiction, it is crucial to acknowledge the possible dysfunction in the addict's biology as it may influence treatment.

Cognitive Distortions

Perhaps the most accepted idea regarding the etiology of sexual addiction is the presence of cognitive distortions. Through past trauma, violence, or pain, the sex addict has formed cognitive distortions about him- or herself—thoughts such as feeling worthless, a negative view of the world, fear or distrust of others, poor self-esteem/self-image, or the idea that sex can alleviate all problems. Sex addicts will have problems separating their feelings from their cognitive distortions. They will seek relationships or situations that are used to prove their cognitive distortions, as in a self-fulfilling prophecy, for example, thinking they are unworthy of a trusting, loving, and committed relationship by taking on casual relationships that will not last.

The sex addict will also have feelings of guilt in respect to his or her unhealthy sexual behavior or guilt from hurting the ones he or she loves by lying, cheating, and/or deceiving, especially when in a committed relationship. Each time the sex addict is confronted with uncomfortable feelings such as sadness, fear, disappointment, or anger, the cognitive distortions resurface. "Pleasure and orgasm is used to soothe and comfort states of internal distress. Sexual feelings merge with shame, sadness, anger, and loneliness, which then become triggers for the addictive cycle."[21] At the peak of the cycle, shame is not felt (escape). Omnipotence, grandiosity, and a false sense of esteem rise up and cover painful experiences of shame. Once the cycle is complete, shame reappears.

Shame is part of the core identity of sex addicts and affects how they view their needs, feelings, and sexuality. These feelings of shame become merged with arousal. The addiction is a metaphor for the unconscious trauma.[22] "Shame and guilt make up the feelings of despair and, when overwhelmed by these emotions, the addict will use the compulsive behavior until the cycle is disrupted and alternative affect coping strategies are established."[23] New holistic techniques for sex addicts to release these feelings of shame are needed in order to replace the sexual behaviors.

Attachment Disorder

Other researchers believe that sexual addiction stems from an attachment disorder. "Sexual addiction is an intimacy disorder that is rooted in impaired early attachment experiences. This impaired bonding causes the developing self to be shrouded in shame."[24] Sex addicts will blame themselves for their caretaker's inability to nurture them, thus producing their initial shame. Their ability to trust is limited, and along with it, the ability for them to bond with others in committed relationships. They often feel that they deserve the worst; that they are not worthy of being cared for or having their needs met. Sex addicts do not have a internal working model of healthy relationships. "As children, when there is a failure in early developmental caretaking, the child is unable to soothe his or her feelings of loneliness, sadness, anger, and fear."[25] The pain caused by the lack of attachment from the caretaker, the original shame, is learned to be soothed through external sexual actions, which then produce shame from the act of the soothing behavior.

Fantasies can also be implemented into the addiction behavior cycle. They give the illusion of an "ideal metaphor" of a relationship. As the sex addict is known to have limited trust in others, having the fantasy gives him or her the illusion of a no-fail relationship. "Real relationships" end up being unequal, as the sex addict partner cannot reciprocate trust and has a fear of disappointment from the other party. "Attachment formation supports the hypothesis that sexual addicts compensate for their inability to form close attachments by fantasizing or yearning about metaphoric surrogates."[26]

Emotional Pain/Trauma

For individuals who have experienced past trauma such as rape, molestation, physical/emotional/sexual abuse, or the death of a loved one, that trauma can potentially manifest in sexual addiction. Individuals who have had past traumatic experiences might engage in self-destructive behaviors to cope with or avoid painful emotions associated with the trauma. For instance, some sex addicts will masturbate constantly as it is a reliable source of relief from emotional pain, loneliness, anxiety, and emptiness.[27] Additionally, sex addicts are sensitive to emotional stimuli and respond intensely. If the sex addict experiences loneliness, the emotion is more intense for the sex addict than a nonaddict; therefore, the intensity enables his or her addiction as it encourages maladaptive coping strategies.[28]

Screening

Knowledge of the screening process is crucial when identifying sex addiction. Additionally, those who suffer from sex addiction may not identify it or may exhibit denial about their addiction. Statements by sex addicts that convey their denial will be similar to the following: "I am not oversexed. I deserve it," "Just one more time won't hurt," and/or "It isn't so bad since everyone does it."[29] Counselors must be ready and expect to hear those words from the sex addict.

In the process of screening those who have sex addiction from those who do not, awareness of what constitutes addictive behaviors will assist in the process. The sex addict will display a pattern of an inability to control his or her behavior, have serious consequences due to his or her behavior, display an obsession with sexual activities and fantasies as a primary coping strategy, present a change in mood when engaging in such activities, have difficulty functioning socially, occupationally, and recreationally, and spend an inordinate amount of time engaging in sexual activities.[30]

There are a number of assessment tools available to identify sex addiction:

- The Sexual Dependency Inventory-Revised (SDI-R) is a reliable and valid assessment in identifying different categories of sex addiction, including fantasy, seductive role-playing, voyeurism, exhibitionism, paying/trading for sex, pain exchange, intrusive sex, exploitive sex, and anonymous sex. The SDI-R is best for distinguishing the sex addict from the nonaddict.[31]

- The Sex Addiction Screening Test-Revised (SAST-R) is designed to identify sexually compulsive or addictive behavior. Preoccupation (obsessive thoughts about sexual behavior), loss of control (inability to stop behavior), relationship disturbance (sexual behavior negatively

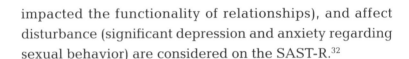

impacted the functionality of relationships), and affect disturbance (significant depression and anxiety regarding sexual behavior) are considered on the SAST-R.[32]

- The Compulsive Sexual Disorder Interview (CSDI) by Black and Kehrberg analyzes the compulsions and enables professionals to get an overall picture of why addicts engage in their compulsions. The CSDI includes a description of cognitions and behaviors involved in the sex addict's behaviors and identifies the impairments reported.[33]

- The Sexual History Questionnaire (SHQ) by Gaither and Sellbom is beneficial to assess any sexual behavior such as oral, vaginal, anal intercourse, and masturbation occurring within three months.

- Professionals interested in measuring sexual aggression between men and women should utilize the Aggressive Sexual Behavior Inventory (ASBI) as it identifies sexual force, alcohol and other drugs, verbal manipulation, callous sexual attitudes, and violence.[34]

The aforementioned assessment instruments can be helpful for professionals to identify and understand the sex addict's behaviors. Additionally, their use can provide insight for the therapeutic relationship and for the addict as he or she learns more about the disease of addiction. Identifying the sex addict's thought patterns is also an important component of the screening process. The sex addict's thought process may be irrational, illogical, and unfounded. Furthermore, the sex addict is likely to have feelings of shame and guilt; therefore, a consideration of those particular emotions should be part of the screening process.

Moreover, gathering information regarding the time of onset, history, duration, frequency, and the progression of addiction is important as it enables the sex addict to receive an individualized treatment plan and gives counselors a better understanding of the addict's addiction.[35] Understanding the different types of behaviors and thought processes reveals how the sex addict functions with his or her addiction. Lastly, the most important aspect of the screening process is identifying if the sex addict is ready to change since the desire to change is essential for success of the therapeutic relationship.

Diagnosing

The *DSM-IV-TR* does not classify obsessive-compulsive sexual behaviors as addiction. The sexual disorders in the *DSM-IV-TR* focus on deficiencies in sexual activity such as female orgasmic disorder and hypoactive sexual desire disorder. *Paraphilia* is a disorder stated in the *DSM-IV-TR* that somewhat resembles sex addiction as types of paraphilia could be considered as dissociative/coping behaviors for sex addiction. Paraphilia includes exhibitionism, fetishism, frotteurism, pedophilia, sexual masochism, sexual sadism, transvestic fetishism, and voyeurism. Although obsessive-compulsive sexual behaviors are not characterized as addiction in the *DSM-IV-TR*, commonalities are present with substance dependence as sex addicts also experience tolerance, withdrawal, loss of control, and adverse consequences.[36]

Criteria

A set of established criteria help to clearly diagnose sexual addiction. The first three criteria must be present in order for someone to be diagnosed with sexual addiction:

A. Failure to resist the urge to act out in a sexual behavior.

B. The presence of tension or anxiety before and following the sexual behavior.

C. A sense of euphoria or numbness (relief) at the time of the sexual behavior.

At least five of the following criteria must be witnessed or reported. In sexual addiction, as in all manifestations of addiction, there is a frequent preoccupation with their sexual behavior and/or an obsession of sexual thoughts as a means to cope with life's problems and negative feelings. "There are some self-identified sex addicts who rarely act out behaviorally."[37]

This preoccupation causes disruption in their lives by redirecting all energies on completing ritual behaviors. A majority of time will be spent on these ritualistic activities prior, during, and after the sexual behavior. The frequency of their sexual behaviors will increase over time and will often continue longer than intended. Sexual behaviors take center stage while daily activities (social, academic, work, and hobbies) progressively assume a lower priority. A tolerance or need to intensify/increase the sexual behavior will build in order to receive the same effect of euphoria or numbness. Cravings, obsessive thoughts about sex or sexual acts/aversions, compulsive behaviors, fantasies, and withdrawal symptoms soon appear and increase as the tolerance builds. Efforts to decrease, manage, or discontinue the sexual behavior are unsuccessful or are able to be maintained for a limited time with return to use.

Sexual behaviors continue despite problems created by the sex addict's preoccupation or unhealthy sexual behaviors. Physically, the sex addict can place him- or herself in danger of sexually transmitted diseases and physically harmful situations, including physical violence or rape as related to his or her exhibitionism. Legal problems can also arise as a result of the behaviors, such as charges of sexual harassment (flashing), prostitution, stalking, voyeurism, exhibitionism, rape, incest, or child molestation. Sex addicts can suffer financially due to their preoccupation with sexual acts. They can lose their job, create debt from their behaviors such as prostitution or purchase of sexual aids like pornography, phone sex, prostitution, and even divorce if the person is in a committed relationship. The sex addict can also suffer spiritually.[38] Following is the outlined criteria for a sexual addiction diagnosis. The reported symptoms must be present for a period of *at least* one month or present intermittently over a long period of time.

Diagnosis of Sexual Addiction[39]

A. Recurrent failure to resist impulses to engage in a specified sexual behavior.

B. Increasing sense of tension immediately prior to initiating the sexual behavior.

C. Pleasure or relief at the time of engaging in the sexual behavior.

D. At least five of the following:

    1. Frequent preoccupation with the sexual behavior or with activity that is preparatory to the sexual behavior.

    2. Frequent engaging in the sexual behavior to a greater extent or over a longer period than intended.

    3. Repeated efforts to reduce, control, or stop the sexual behavior.

    4. A great deal of time spent in activities necessary for the sexual behavior, engaging in the sexual behavior, or recovering from its effects.

    5. Frequent engaging in the sexual behavior when expected to fulfill occupational, academic, domestic, or social obligations.

    6. Important social, occupational, or recreational activities given up or reduced because of the sexual behavior.

    7. Continuation of the sexual behavior despite knowledge of having persistent or recurrent social, financial, psychological, or physical problems that are caused or exacerbated by the sexual behavior.

    8. Tolerance: need to increase the intensity or frequency of the sexual behavior in order to achieve the desired effect, or diminished effect with continued sexual behavior of the same intensity.

    9. Restlessness or irritability if unable to engage in the sexual behavior.

10. Some symptoms of the disturbance have persisted for at least one month or have occurred repeatedly over a longer period of time.

Following the diagnosis and screening process, the therapeutic relationship can begin. The therapeutic relationship is a partnership between a counselor and the client in the development of goals and treatment plan. When the sex addict is part of the goal development, he or she is more likely to be motivated in his or her recovery. Therapy is crucial to sex addicts as it aids them to cope with the etiology of their disease, learn about their behaviors, assist in their understanding of their behavior, and determine positive behaviors to counteract the enabling behaviors. The therapeutic relationship is an opportunity for the sex addict to learn how to develop intimacy in a nonsexual setting, experience a relationship without manipulation, and increase self-esteem and build a healthy self-concept. Confrontation is not advised during the therapeutic relationship as it may be counterproductive. Confrontation could possibly be a reenactment of abuse to the sexual addict; therefore, creating negative feelings such as shame and guilt.[40]

There are several theories which professionals can work from that benefit the therapeutic process. Individual psychotherapy, cognitive behavioral therapy, and medication are useful when treating sexual addiction.[41]

Theories and Treatment

Motivational Interviewing

The therapeutic alliance between the sex addict and the therapist is crucial for the success of treatment and recovery. Progression and development of the alliance ensures the sex addict remain in therapy in which recovery is probable, as a number of studies have demonstrated a link between the quality of the therapeutic alliance and outcome of treatment.

Additionally, motivational interviewing fosters motivation and change in resistant clients by utilizing reflecting listening techniques, in which the therapist echoes what the client conveys from a neutral standpoint. Motivational interviewing is a tool for therapists to develop a strong relationship with their clients without the clients becoming dependent on them. Shame and unworthiness are major issues sex addicts experience. Motivational interviewing can assist clients to overcome their negative emotions and emphasize self-efficacy, which improves their internal locus of control and affirmations that reinforce the sex addict's positive qualities.[42] Incorporating motivational interviewing with different theories is possible and increases the probability of success in the therapeutic relationship.

Cognitive Behavioral Theory (CBT)

Sex addiction involves cognitive distortions, unmanageability, ritualization, fantasy, euphoric recall, preoccupation, guilt, and shame.[43] While developing a therapeutic trust with the sexual addict, professionals can assist in his or her recovery by identifying triggers and brainstorm how to cope with such triggers. Professionals can identify the sex addiction behaviors and how they facilitate maladaptive behaviors and/or emotions. Psychoeducation pertaining to intimacy and the differences between degrading and enriching sex can benefit the therapeutic process. Examples of CBT strategies are forming an abstinence contract, carrying an index card with therapeutic phrases or sentences, changing negative self-talk to positive self-talk, counteracting irrational thoughts, and relapse prevention.

Object Relations Theory

Object relations is considered a developmental theory in which it is essential during the therapeutic relationship for the therapist to identify the client's developmental deficits and characterological needs. In order for the sex addict to attain a long-term change and be successful in his or her recovery, an integration of the assessment of the stages in object relations theory, cognitive distortion, behavior interventions, and transference relationship are needed. There are four stages in the object relations theory and each are explained in relation to sex addiction, providing a different perspective on treating sex addiction. According to Parker and Guest, all sexually addicted clients are developmentally deficient in one or more of the following stages:[44]

1. **Autistic Stage**

   When the sex addict experiences a deficiency in this stage, he or she is more likely to have trouble forming attachments. Dissociation is a coping mechanism for sex addicts when they have an inability to develop meaningful relationships. Dissociative behaviors enable sex addicts to avoid contact with another human being, and therefore, are more likely to isolate themselves by engaging in Internet pornography, voyeurism, pornography, and masturbation. If the individual has issues that stemmed from the autistic stage, it is therapeutic to focus on strategies to cope with anxiety, develop therapeutic bonds, to be in the here and now, and focus on the development of healthy relationships. Focus on interpersonal relationships is crucial as long-term recovery depends on their satisfaction with their relationships with other people.

2. **Symbiotic Stage**

   In relation to sex addiction, those who are incomplete in the symbiotic stage have a major need for attachment and engage in sexual behaviors to avoid feelings of abandonment and shame; therefore, are more likely to engage in prostitution, multiple relationships, and have a love addiction. The therapeutic process should focus on their need for nurturing and to reduce anxiety while developing alternative and healthy ways to get their needs met. A discussion of the loss of their addiction should be part of their recovery.

3. **Separation-Individuation Stage**

The sex addict who experiences an incompletion in this stage is likely to display behavioral traits of narcissism and borderline personality. When the child is separated from his or her parents during the separation-individuation stage, the child is more likely to have a hypersensitivity to criticisms, unconscious dependency needs, and experience inferiority. When experiencing the aforementioned tendencies, the sex addict is more likely to be predatory and need a victim to obtain a feeling of control over his or her inferiority and meet his or her unconscious needs for worthiness. Additionally, the sex addict has a lack of empathy; therefore, engages in multiple affairs with a component of hypersexuality, use of prostitutes, swing parties, and certain forms of pedophilia and incest. Therapists working with the sex addict who displays narcissistic traits may experience a sense of being used and not being seen as an individual; therefore, it is essential for the therapist to remain always in control of the therapeutic relationship. During the therapeutic relationship, it is important to notice if there is a lack of empathy by the client, and mirror the client, finding balance between giving feedback and his or her hypersensitivity to criticism. It is important for the sex addict to acknowledge his or her need for feeling special.

Borderline sex addicts were not allowed to separate from their primary caregiver and are likely to engage in behaviors as a defense against emptiness when experiencing feelings of loneliness. Such individuals have difficulties controlling their impulses and have unstable personal relationships. According to Parker and Guest, they need structure in the therapeutic relationship as they have a tendency to devaluate it. A possible intervention for borderline sex addicts is assisting them to see both the good and bad in people.

A commonality is present in each stage in that clients, who are deficient from a particular stage, experience uncomfortable sensations such as anxiety, fear, depression, and anger. When experiencing those particular sensations, the sex addict acts to shift the mood to a more comfortable state and/or to meet his or her needs. Parker and Guest support the understanding that the function of the sex addict's sexual behavior is crucial for the changes in his or her behavior and sustaining the change.

Shame Reduction

Shame is considered by leading theorists and researchers as the core of sex addiction. A focus on therapeutic intervention with shame is needed by professionals when working with sex addicts. There are steps to reduce shame according to Adams and Robinson:[45]

1. Understand the origin of the shame and its function in the addictive system.

2. Differentiate between shame and guilt.

3. Identify the defenses utilized to deny the painful feelings created by the shame.

4. Utilize specific shame reduction strategies at critical points in the treatment process.

5. Change negative core beliefs that reinforce shame.

As the therapist and client are going through the steps in shame reduction, strategies should also be integrated to ensure its therapeutic value. The therapist should establish rapport, support, encouragement, and understanding of the sex addict. Sex addicts must be educated about how shame enables the maladaptive behaviors in order to cope with the negative feelings. An exploration of shame and how it consists of feelings of inadequacy, unworthiness, mistrust, loneliness, sadness, guilt, and anger must be accomplished to understand its etiology and purpose. Furthermore, shame is part of the core identity of sex addicts in which it affects their needs, feelings, sexuality, and arousal.[46] A focus on the client's strengths and affirmations can be utilized to replace negative feelings and shame.

Creative Modalities

A lack of focus on shame impedes the sex addict's chances of recovery and will lead to regression and relapse. Shame is not an easy subject to discuss and it could be tough for sex addicts to verbalize their shame. Professionals should consider incorporating creative modalities such as art, music, dance, and drama into their practice to assist the sex addict's ability to express and process shame. Art therapy and psychodrama help the sex addict to explore thoughts and feelings such as anger, sadness, and anxieties. For instance, "art materials allow for ventilation and transformation of aggressive and violent emotions previously dealt with by compulsive and out-of-control behaviors."[47]

Narcissism is also present in sex addiction and art therapy is considered nurturing for the narcissistic sex addict. Another creative modality to consider is sandtray therapy. Sandtray therapy facilitates the process of finding meaning, reconstruction of one's inner world, and the resolution of traumatic experiences. Sandtray assists the sex addict to reveal his or her personal world in which the addict's beliefs, values, stories, and feelings are revealed, acknowledged, and validated.[48] Professionals are encouraged to integrate creative modalities with existing techniques as they break down defenses more quickly and less traumatically which could be beneficial for clients who have a tough time expressing themselves.[49]

Group Therapy

In addition to individual counseling, group counseling can provide the sex addict a safe place to express and share his or her feelings. In group counseling, sex addicts have an opportunity to identify with others, access support, and therefore, feel less lonely.[50] Participation in group is an essential aspect of early recovery for the sex addict as it can address sexual acting-out behaviors.[51] Constructive feedback is part of the group process and can assist the sex addict to become aware of irrational thoughts, cognitive distortions, dynamics pertaining to his or her addiction, and maladaptive behaviors. Furthermore, group counseling can teach the sex addict how to develop nonsexual relationships and/or meaningful relationships.

Psychopharmacology

While medication is not typically used with people engaging in maladaptive sexual behavior, it is possible that it can benefit the sex addict. For instance, antidepressants can help decrease the intensity of the sexual experience.[52] Serotonin reuptake blockers cause a reduction in sexual desire and regulate the intensity of orgasm,[53] which can be helpful when treating the sex addict.

Conclusion

Pending the release of the *DSM-5*, current research debunks the misunderstandings surrounding sex addicts and offers adequate criteria regarding a diagnosis of sexual addiction. With the increased attention surrounding sex addiction it is imperative that clinicians today become familiar with the characteristics, etiology, criteria, and treatment of sex addiction. Though there is limited research on the precise treatment needed for sexual addiction, we can utilize the research we have now, as well as information that corresponds to other manifestations of addiction, such as substance abuse and pathological gambling in order to develop strategies for treatment.

5

Eating Disorders

Cortney S. Warren

Emily K. White

Kim Claudat

Holly B. LaPota

Eating pathology and substance use disorders are highly comorbid. As such, researchers and clinicians have proposed various theories to understand how, when, and why these disorders co-occur. The purpose of this chapter is to summarize the literature examining comorbid eating pathology and substance use. Specifically, we review: 1) the diagnostic criteria for the eating and substance use disorders; 2) prevalence data on their comorbidity; 3) three primary theories developed to conceptually understand their co-occurrence; and, 4) practical implications for clinicians who treat this population and researchers.

Diagnostic Descriptions of Eating Pathology and Substance Use Disorders

Eating Pathology

Eating disorders (EDs) are among the most common yet serious psychological problems facing females in the United States today. EDs and eating pathology—a term used to describe eating disorder symptoms not specific to one disorder—are characterized by maladaptive attitudes, behaviors, and intrapsychic experiences around eating, weight, and body image that cause significant distress or impairment. According to the most recent edition of the *Diagnostic and Statistical Manual of Mental Disorders, Text-Revision (DSM-IV-TR)*, EDs fall into three primary categories: anorexia nervosa (AN), bulimia nervosa (BN), and eating disorder not otherwise specified (EDNOS).[1]

AN is characterized by a significant disturbance in the perception of body shape or size (e.g., seeing one's body as physically larger than it is); an intense fear of gaining weight; refusal to maintain a minimally normal body weight (i.e., less than 85 percent of what is expected for one's age and height); and the loss of menses (in women who are postmenarcheal and not taking an oral contraceptive). Individuals with AN are preoccupied with attaining and maintaining an extremely thin body, which leads them to become dangerously underweight. AN has two primary subtypes that indicate the presence or absence of regular binge eating or purging: the restricting subtype (AN-R) describes individuals who severely restrict food intake (only) whereas the binge-eating/purging subtype (AN-BP) describes individuals who restrict food intake but also regularly engage in binge eating or purging episodes (described and defined below).

Like AN, BN is characterized by an overvaluation of weight and shape (i.e., placing high importance on physical appearance as a determinant of personal worth) and an excessive drive for thinness. However, BN is also characterized by recurrent binge eating episodes followed by inappropriate compensatory methods to prevent weight gain. Binge eating is defined as eating a significantly larger amount of food than most individuals would eat under similar circumstances in a short amount of time (e.g., less than two hours) while feeling loss of control over what and how much is eaten. Additionally, binge eating usually continues until an individual is uncomfortably full and is commonly associated with profound feelings of shame, anxiety, and sadness. To compensate for the calories consumed during recurrent binge eating episodes, individuals with BN engage in compensatory behaviors such as self-induced vomiting, misuse of laxatives or diuretics, fasting, or intensive exercise. The *DSM-IV-TR* specifies two subtypes of BN to identify the compensatory methods used: the purging subtype (BN-P) describes individuals who regularly engage in self-induced vomiting or the misuse of purgative agents (e.g., laxatives, diuretics, enemas, diet pills) whereas the nonpurging subtype (BN-NP) describes individuals whose compensatory behavior does not involve ingestion or manipulation of a substance (e.g., excessive exercising, caloric restriction, fasting). To meet the criteria for BN, an individual cannot currently meet the diagnostic criteria for AN, and individuals with BN are generally normal weight or overweight.

Finally, EDNOS is a catch-all diagnostic category used to diagnose disorders of eating, weight, and body image that do not meet diagnostic criteria for AN or BN. For example, a patient who regularly menstruates but meets all other diagnostic criteria for AN would receive a diagnosis of EDNOS. Similarly, a patient of normal body weight who regularly uses inappropriate compensatory behavior after eating an amount of food that is not considered a binge (e.g., self-induced vomiting after consuming two cookies) would be diagnosed with EDNOS.

The most commonly researched subcategory of EDNOS is binge eating disorder (BED), which is a provisional diagnosis in the *DSM-IV-TR* and is likely to be added to the upcoming *DSM-5*.[2] BED is characterized by recurrent episodes of binge eating with an absence of compensatory weight-control behaviors. In BED, binge eating episodes are markedly distressing and characterized by eating more rapidly than normal; eating until uncomfortably full; eating when not hungry; eating alone due to embarrassment around the quantity one eats; and feeling intense guilt, disgust, or depression after eating. Dissatisfaction with body shape and appearance is common in individuals with BED;[3] but unlike patients with AN or BN, patients with BED also tend to overeat during normal meals and are often overweight or obese.

Approximately 90 percent of people who suffer from AN and BN are women and girls living in Western cultural contexts.[4] The age of onset is generally during adolescence to young adulthood. The lifetime prevalence of AN is estimated to be 0.5 to 1 percent of women in the United States; for BN, estimates range from 1 to 3 percent.[5] Although the prevalence of BED is not yet well established, research suggests that 5 to 10 percent of individuals seeking treatment for obesity meet criteria for BED, and lifetime prevalence rates are estimated to be about 5 percent in the general population.[6] Notably, the gender disparity is less pronounced in BED: estimates suggest that nearly one-third of BED patients are male.[7]

Substance Use Disorders

As presented in the *DSM-IV-TR*, substance use disorders (SUDs) fall under two main categories: substance abuse and substance dependence. According to the *DSM-IV-TR*, both substance abuse and dependence can be applied to various legal and illegal drugs including (but not limited to) alcohol, nicotine, amphetamines, caffeine, cannabis, cocaine, hallucinogens, opioids, anxiolytics, and phencyclidine. During both substance abuse and dependence, an individual continues to use despite experiencing adverse consequences and significant distress or impairment as a result of his or her substance use.

Substance abuse is characterized by repeated use of a substance despite recurrent negative consequences related to its use. The pattern of maladaptive substance use must be present for at least twelve months and have resulted in at least one of the following impairing conditions: 1) an inability to fulfill obligations at home, school, or work; 2) recurrent legal problems; 3) significant interpersonal problems; or 4) continued use even in dangerous situations that pose imminent threat to the user.

In contrast, substance dependence is considered more severe and is distinguished from substance abuse by the presence of significant physiological, cognitive, and behavioral symptoms that develop from recurrent use.[8] Physiological symptoms include tolerance, which occurs when increased amounts of a substance are needed to induce the same effect, and withdrawal, which refers to the experience of adverse symptoms related to the cessation or reduction of substance use. Individuals struggling with substance dependence often report preoccupying cognitions and ruminative thinking about the substance (e.g., "When can I next use" or "Where am I am going to get my next fix") and a strong drive or "craving" for the substance. Behavioral symptoms include spending a significant amount of time securing the substance, using the substance, or recovering from its effects.

According to the *DSM-IV-TR*, adults between the ages of eighteen and twenty-four have the highest prevalence of SUDs. For example, in 2007, 9 percent of Americans over age twelve (i.e., about 22.3 million individuals) were classified as meeting diagnostic criteria for either substance abuse or dependence over the past year. The majority of these individuals (approximately 70 percent) abused or were dependent on alcohol only; 16 percent used or abused an illicit drug other than alcohol; and 14 percent used alcohol and another illicit substance concomitantly.[9]

Comorbid Eating Pathology and Substance Use Disorders

A large body of research suggests that EDs and SUDs co-occur at rates higher than would be expected in the general population.[10] Epidemiological data suggests that up to 50 percent of women with EDs abuse substances and nearly 35 percent of women with a SUD have an ED.[11] The co-prevalence is bidirectional such that women who seek treatment for EDs exhibit higher rates of substance use than controls[12] and women who seek treatment for SUDs display higher rates of disordered eating than controls.[13] Elevated co-prevalence rates are also echoed in nonclinical samples: Women with subthreshold eating pathology are more likely to use substances[14] and subthreshold substance abusers are more likely to exhibit disordered eating.[15] As such, the research literature generally examines co-prevalence from two perspectives: 1) patients with EDs who use substances and 2) patients with SUDs who exhibit eating pathology.

Substance Use in Patients with Eating Pathology

The National Center on Addiction and Substance Abuse (CASA) estimates that approximately half of women with eating pathology abuse substances; however, data from clinical samples suggest somewhat lower rates. Studies on individuals with BN suggest that approximately 20 to 25 percent drink alcohol,[16] use illicit substances (currently or in the past),[17] and report substance abuse.[18] Co-prevalence rates for individuals with AN are lower, ranging from no substance use to almost 20 percent[19] (with an average estimate of about 10 percent[20]). Given that individuals with AN severely restrict their caloric intake, it is not surprising that they do not use substances with the frequency of those with BN. However, several studies suggest that substance use does occur in individuals with AN, particularly around weight-loss promoting substances.[21]

With regard to symptom presentation, the majority of research suggests that individuals who engage in binge eating and/or purging behavior (e.g., individuals with BN or AN-BP) report more substance use than individuals who present with restrictive symptoms (e.g., individuals with AN-R).[22] For example, Walsh and colleagues found that individuals with AN-BP had rates of substance abuse, alcohol abuse or dependence, and tobacco use that were twice as high as women with AN-R.[23] Additionally, some research suggests that women with EDs are at increased risk for developing SUDs over time. A nine year longitudinal study, for example, found that about 18 percent of women with AN and 30 percent of women with BN developed a SUD.[24] This leads some researchers to suggest that disordered eating may be a risk factor for SUDs (discussed in the "Theories of Causal Etiology" section).[25]

Eating Pathology in Patients with Substance Use Disorders

Overall, women with SUDs report higher rates of eating pathology than nonsubstance users.[26] In a study of 204 women receiving inpatient treatment for SUDs, lifetime prevalence of an ED was 20 percent and the presence of eating pathology was predictive of lower treatment success and increased relapse potential.[27] Similarly, in a sample of thirty-one women enrolled in an alcohol treatment unit (both inpatient and outpatient), about 25 percent were diagnosed with an ED and 33 percent reported engaging in binge eating in the past twenty-eight days.[28] In Holderness and colleagues' review of the comorbidity literature, the authors concluded that a substantial proportion of substance abusers reported a history of BN or other purging-related disorders,[29] with a median lifetime prevalence rate of approximately 20 percent.[30] This is higher than what is typically found for restrictive eating behaviors, the prevalence of which is under 10 percent in individuals with SUDs. Practically, this means that nearly one in five individuals seeking treatment for a SUD will endorse current or historic eating pathology, most often characterized by binge eating and purging-related symptoms (i.e., those related to BN and AN-BP).

With regard to drug use, it is important to note that women increasingly report weight loss as a primary reason to use legal and illegal drugs.[31] In a large sample of 3,305 high school seniors, for example, female cigarette smokers reported significantly greater use of diet pills and amphetamines to lose weight than nonsmoking females.[32] Similarly, a recent study examining methamphetamine use in a sample of 350 adults found that women were five times more likely to attribute initial drug use to a desire to lose weight than men.[33] Furthermore, qualitative studies examining female stimulant users indicate that the rapid, significant weight loss achieved with stimulants is highly reinforcing and is often a primary motivator for continued substance use.[34] Consequently, when considering drug use aimed at weight loss (which is frequently seen in individuals with BN), the diagnostic overlap is likely higher than current estimates suggest for women.

Limitations of Existing Research

There are various limitations of the extant co-prevalence research. Existing research rarely differentiates between the various forms of SUDs (i.e., substance abuse versus substance dependence) or specifies the particular substance used.[35] Alhough eating pathology appears to co-occur less frequently with illicit substances than with alcohol or nicotine, emerging research suggests high comorbidity between eating pathology and drugs with weight-loss side effects, which makes knowing the type of substance used and motivation for use (e.g., to lose weight, for fun) increasingly important. Additionally, sex differences are infrequently reported in the literature due to a low prevalence base-rate of EDs in men. However, the prevalence of SUDs is high among men and limited research suggests that men with BED are more likely to report lifetime SUDs than women with BED.[36] Continued research on these relationships in men is needed.

Eating Pathology and Substance Use/Abuse: Conceptual and Etiological Overlap

Most theories attempting to understand the high levels of comorbidity between EDs and SUDs propose a co-prevalence framework, which posits that there is an etiological or causal relationship between the two groups of disorders. The most popular theories can be divided into three primary categories: 1) eating pathology as a process or behavioral addiction;

2) shared etiological theories; and 3) causal etiological theories. Conceptual and empirical support for each category emerges from biological, psychological, and/or socially-based sources.

Eating Pathology as a Process Addiction

One prominent conceptualization proposes that EDs are best conceptualized as addictive disorders. While the term is not currently defined in an existing diagnostic manual, addiction is typically used to describe substance dependence as it is defined in the *DSM-IV-TR*. In this context and colloquially, the term addiction is used to describe a pattern of behavioral, physiological, and cognitive symptoms that develop due to substance use characterized by tolerance to the effects of the substance; withdrawal symptoms that develop when use of the substance is terminated; and continued use of the substance despite adverse consequences.

Although addiction generally refers to the abuse of substances that affect the central nervous system (e.g., alcohol, nicotine, cocaine), researchers postulate that a number of behavioral syndromes function as addictions because of their resemblance to psychoactive substance dependence.[37] As defined by Goodman, a behavioral or process addiction can be defined as recurrent behavior used to yield pleasure and/or provide relief from internal discomfort that an individual is unable to control or stop despite significant adverse consequences.[38] Using this broader definition of addiction, a number of behavioral syndromes can manifest as process addictions, including pathological gambling, sexual activity (e.g., engaging in sex, watching pornography), computer/Internet use, shopping, and eating.

Research support for this theory stems from the behavioral similarities between the SUDs and EDs (e.g., antecedents of substance use/behavior, experience of substance use/behavior). A large body of research focuses on the similarity between binge drinking and binge eating and/or purging (e.g., in BN or AN-BP). For example, binge eating and drinking share common characteristics, including preoccupying thoughts about the substance or behavior; craving for the substance or behavior; a repeated urge to use the substance or engage in the behavior despite negative consequences; a loss of control over the substance or behavior; repeated failed attempts to stop using the substance or engaging in the behavior; and the use of the substance or behavior to temporarily regulate emotions and relieve negative affect.[39] Withdrawal symptoms are also similar: patients actively trying to stop binge eating and those who stop using a substance commonly report symptoms like poor concentration, irritability, restlessness, moodiness, anxiety, migraines, insomnia, and lethargy.[40]

Also in support of this theory, research suggests that individuals suffering from EDs and SUDs often use food or drugs to alleviate affective symptoms that are causing distress. Individuals with EDs and SUDs report high rates of anxiety, depression, and other psychosocial problems.[41] As such, individuals may eat or use substances in response to emotional stress, loneliness, or interpersonal conflict. This often evolves into a cycle of coping with negative affect using maladaptive behavior (e.g., substance use, binge eating) that, in turn, causes increased negative affect. For example, individuals with SUDs often feel temporary relief from negative affect during substance use but increased guilt after use.[42] Similarly, engaging in binge eating and purging behavior temporarily reduces anxiety and tension for most individuals with an ED, but is quickly followed by negative affect or guilt after engaging in the behavior.[43]

Theories of Shared Etiology

A second primary theoretical framework proposes that a third, predisposing factor contributes to the onset of both EDs and SUDs. From this conceptualization, researchers posit that biological and genetic factors (e.g., physiological functioning, shared genetic material, family history of EDs and/or substance abuse) account for the co-prevalence of these disorders. In support of the shared etiological perspective, genetic research suggests that BN and drug use have some familial heritability. In one study, for example, nearly 83 percent of the correlation between BN and illicit drug use was accounted for by shared genetic factors.[44] Also in support of this theory is research suggesting that the brain's reward system is activated by psychoactive substances and behavioral processes in similar ways.[45] For example, obese individuals who engage in binge eating display many of the same reward processes in the brain as substance abusers who engage in drug use.[46] While specific candidate genes have not been identified to date, it is possible that a shared genetic vulnerability to both EDs and SUDs accounts for the co-occurrence of these disorders.

The shared etiological theory is also supported by some research investigating personality style as a predictor of behavior (e.g., impulsivity, sensation seeking). Many researchers posit that individuals who have high trait impulsivity and heightened sensation seeking may be more likely to engage in both substance use and bulimic-type behaviors. Specifically, individuals with heightened reward sensitivity are more likely to act on cravings, whether those cravings are to binge eat or to use drugs.[47] As such, some clinicians and researchers prefer to conceptualize individuals who engage in substance abuse, binge eating, and other addiction-like behaviors (e.g., sex, gambling) as individuals with addictive personalities. In this way, treatment providers focus on the character of the person rather than the actual substance or behavior that appears most problematic at any given time.[48]

Finally, sociocultural data examining the role of familial relationships, peer interactions, and cultural environment lends some support for the shared etiological perspective. Family history studies suggest that an individual is at increased risk for developing a substance use disorder if one immediate family member has a history of the same problem.[49] For example, one study suggested that offspring of individuals with a history of illicit substance use (including opioids, cocaine, and/or cannabis) were at an eight-times greater risk for developing a drug use disorder.[50] Research also suggests that having a first-degree relative with a history of alcoholism is related to more severe eating pathology and substance use behaviors.[51] Similarly, there is an increased risk of developing an ED if a first-degree relative suffers from an ED.[52] Although these data are also used to demonstrate a shared genetic predisposition for EDs and SUDs, the general nature of the family environment appears to have a direct influence on the development of both substance use and EDs.[53] For example, a family environment characterized by high expressed emotion,[54] high levels of criticism,[55] and significant amounts of conflict between family members[56] puts children at risk for the later development of an ED. Consequently, according to this theory, a genetic heritability risk combined with a negative, emotionally-labile family environment and specific personality disposition can cause an individual to develop a comorbid ED and SUD.

Theories of Causal Etiology

A third explanatory framework suggests that mental illness in one area increases an individual's risk for developing problems in many other areas. Typically, causal etiological theories presume that an ED is initially present, which increases the chance of other pathology, including SUDs.[57] These theories emerged because there was little empirical support for initial substance abuse developing into disordered eating, but a moderate amount of data suggesting that disordered eating predisposes someone to develop a substance abuse problem.

Support for causal etiological theories emerges from biological research investigating physiological correlates of food deprivation and addiction withdrawal. For instance, numerous reviews outline the rewarding effects of food within the dopaminergic system of the brain, especially after a period of deprivation.[58] Engaging in restrictive eating (and therefore entering a state of food deprivation) may alter the dopaminergic reward system such that it leads to increased consumption of alternative reinforcing substances, like alcohol or other drugs.[59] Additionally, operant learning paradigms suggest that reducing the reinforcing value of food may lead to increases in the reinforcing value of other alternatives.[60] For instance, research using animals (e.g., rats, mice) demonstrates that food deprivation leads to increased use of various substances, including alcohol, tobacco, cocaine, and opioid-type substances.[61] When examined in humans, however, the findings are less clear. One study comparing alcohol use in individuals with BN to healthy controls after a period of food deprivation found no significant differences between the two groups.[62] However, other research suggests that chronic dieting is related to increased alcohol consumption in women[63] and that food deprivation increases nicotine intake in food-deprived women.[64]

Additional support for this theory comes from the common clinical observation that many individuals in remission from a SUD develop eating pathology and vice versa, thereby "replacing" one addictive substance for another. For example, women may replace one ineffective coping mechanism (i.e., binge eating) with another (i.e., binge drinking) if the initial coping method is no longer available.[65] An interesting case study documented an extreme fluctuation between symptoms of BN and alcoholism in a male patient who developed symptoms of BN only when abstinent from alcohol.[66] Furthermore, once he resumed drinking, the bulimic symptoms ceased.

Limitations of Existing Theories

While numerous theories try to explain the etiological connection between EDs and SUDs, little research extends beyond merely examining the nature of co-prevalence. Currently, the field is lacking theories that sufficiently explain the functional relationship between eating pathology and SUDs. Additionally, many studies contain critical methodological weaknesses that limit the generalization of their findings (see Holderness et al., 1994 for a review).[67] For instance, the primary constructs of what constitutes an eating or substance use disorder are not consistently defined (e.g., researchers disagree about the amount of food or drug that constitutes a binge). Additionally, very few existing studies include control samples for comparison; many samples are treatment-seeking (as opposed to community samples); and, much of this research is decades old based on outdated criteria from previous versions of the *DSM* (some of which differ significantly from the current *DSM-IV-TR*).

Eating Pathology and Substance Use: Practical Implications

Various factors should be considered when treating someone with a comorbid ED and SUD. First, a thorough risk assessment should be conducted upon admission for treatment because these individuals often present with more severe symptoms than individuals with a single diagnosis.[68] For example, a higher incidence of past drug use was found in a small sample of patients who died due to an ED.[69] In another study, individuals diagnosed with an ED who reported past suicide attempts also reported frequent past drug use.[70] When conducting the assessment, it is useful to evaluate the presence of substance use and eating pathology through a thorough diagnostic interview with the patient and with a third party to corroborate the information.[71]

Second, treatment providers should be aware that past eating pathology may emerge during and following substance detoxification.[72] Women who seek treatment for EDs exhibit higher rates of substance use than controls[73] and women who seek treatment for substance abuse display higher rates of disordered eating than controls. Consequently, as the SUD is treated, eating pathology may emerge more strongly even if it was in remission prior to the current admission. This process is sometimes referred to as addiction transfer.[74] When this occurs, it should be addressed directly and quickly. Furthermore, individuals in recovery from SUDs often gain large amounts of weight following substance cessation.[75] Consequently, during treatment and throughout the recovery process, eating pathology should be monitored because individuals with greater appearance satisfaction exhibit lower relapse rates[76] and because individuals with preexisting body image concerns may experience symptom exacerbation if they gain weight during treatment. Preparing clients for this change and providing preventive health-related counseling (e.g., around nutrition, exercise) may help to alleviate some of their concerns.

Third, treatment providers should be aware that some classes of substances have clear weight-related side effects. Historically, stimulants (e.g., amphetamines) were used to treat severe forms of obesity in the United States. While their use for weight loss is no longer indicated by the Food and Drug Administration (FDA), stimulants continue to be commonly abused for their pleasurable side effects (e.g., increased energy, enhanced alertness, decreased appetite, weight loss, euphoria).[77] The weight-loss side effects associated with stimulants also make this class of drugs particularly appealing to women with high weight and shape concerns, such as those with eating pathology.[78] As previously discussed, substance abusers increasingly report weight-loss as a primary reason for initiating and continuing drug use[79] and this finding is quite robust for stimulants (e.g., methamphetamine).[80] Furthermore, some legal substances (e.g., diet pills, over-the-counter medications) mimic the effects of illegal stimulants; therefore, the use of these substances is often elevated in individuals with a strong desire to lose weight.[81] When individuals report weight-loss as a motivation for initiating or continuing substance use, treatment providers need to address these concerns to effectively treat the SUD.

Fourth, individuals with co-occurring EDs and SUDs may present with other psychiatric and personality disorders, such as major depressive disorder, post-traumatic stress disorder, borderline personality disorder, and impulse control disorders.[82] Given the complications that may arise when any of these disorders are present, attention to interactions between symptom clusters will be critical to effectively treat comorbid conditions.

Finally, addiction treatment programs that address both disorders concurrently likely have the greatest chance of success. Individuals in substance abuse treatment who exhibit eating pathology should participate in supplemental individual psychotherapy with an emphasis on food consumption, body image enhancement, and meal planning (in addition to the general substance abuse treatment protocol).[83] For example, Lindsay and colleagues recently developed a twelve-week supplemental health and body image curriculum designed for women in substance abuse treatment who report weight concerns called Healthy Steps to Freedom (HSF).[84] Outcome data from 124 adult women recruited from substance abuse treatment facilities revealed that eating pathology significantly decreased after HSF program participation whereas health-related behaviors (e.g., increased healthy food consumption) and knowledge (e.g., understanding of basic nutrition, exercise) increased. Supplemental programs like HSF serve to provide integrative treatment to individuals with comorbid SUDs and eating pathology. If not using a structured programmatic supplement, specific topics that a treatment provider may want to address with patients include motivation for substance use, coping with emotion, managing interpersonal stress, reward sensitivity, family dynamics around eating and substance use, body image, and impulse control.[85]

6

Impulse Control Disorders

Lesley Dickson, MD

Impulse Control Disorders Not Classified Elsewhere are a group of psychiatric disorders characterized by a repeated inability to resist the urge to engage in a behavior or resist an impulse or drive to perform an act that is harmful to the person or to others. Additionally, there is a sense of increasing tension prior to the act that is followed by a sense of relief, usually short-lived, subsequent to performance of the act. Presently, there are five named disorders of impulse in *DSM-IV-TR*, which include pathological gambling, intermittent explosive disorder, pyromania, kleptomania, and trichotillomania in addition to impulse control disorder not otherwise specified. There are other proposed disorders of impulse, but they have names such as compulsive sexual behavior and compulsive buying, leading to the question of the relationship of compulsive to impulsive behaviors. Two other important questions are whether they are similar enough to addictive disorders to be classified together and do they share the same underlying pathologies.

Impulsivity is a personality trait characterized by a predisposition toward rapid and unplanned reactions or actions in response to external or internal stimuli.[1] The individual typically acts without regard to the potential outcome and consequences of the action and fails to consider the impact on him- or herself or others, including possible legal consequences. Impulsivity is found in many psychiatric diagnoses and in its milder forms can be a contribution to the extroverted personality who is popular at parties and other social events. Impulsivity is also characteristic of many who become addicted to substances and those who seek intense external stimuli. The disorders with names such as compulsive buying and compulsive sexual behavior are also characterized by repetitive and damaging behaviors and perhaps belong in the same group as impulse control disorders while obsessive-compulsive disorder, characterized by unwanted obsessive thoughts and undesired ritualistic behaviors, is probably very different.

The *DSM-IV-TR* diagnoses of intermittent explosive disorder, kleptomania, pyromania, and trichotillomania will be discussed in this chapter. (See Chapter Three for discussion of pathological gambling.) These four diagnoses are rarely diagnosed and treated in the clinical setting and therefore have been assumed to be infrequent. Additionally, there are few studies that have been conducted that could lead to an understanding of the underlying psychopathology, and few treatment protocols from which to draw recommendations. Much of what is known is drawn from the much more common problem of pathological gambling and then extrapolated to these rarer problems. Following the discussion of the four disorders will be a brief overview of some of the commonalities these disorders share with other addictions, primarily the addiction to substances and how they might explain the impulse control disorders. Also, the proposed changes in *DSM-5* will be described briefly.

Intermittent Explosive Disorder

Individuals with Intermittent Explosive Disorder (IED) fail to resist the urge to engage in aggressive impulses resulting in serious assaults or destruction of property. The degree of aggression is grossly out of proportion to any provocation or psychosocial stressor and the individual may describe a sense of tension or arousal preceding the attack and a sense of relief following the action. The symptoms, often described as spells or attacks, appear within minutes to hours, are usually of short duration and remit spontaneously. Later, there may be a sense of remorse or regret. There are many other diagnoses that must be considered and ruled out before making the diagnosis of IED and they include Antisocial Personality, Borderline Personality, psychotic disorders, a manic episode, conduct disorder, and Attention Deficit Hyperactivity Disorder. Additionally, a medical condition such as head injury or dementia of Alzheimer's disease and the influence of a drug of abuse or some medications must also be considered and eliminated.[2, 3] Therefore the diagnosis of IED is often one of exclusion since aggression is commonly seen in many psychiatric problems.

Those with IED may show other signs of aggressiveness between explosive episodes and the disorder will frequently lead to job loss, school problems, failed relationships, accidents, injuries, and incarcerations. There may be nonspecific findings on EEGs and neuropsychological testing that lead to hypotheses of mild brain damage, which is often supported by nonspecific findings on neurological examination and developmental difficulties. It was originally thought that IED is much more common in males than females, but more recent data indicates a male to female ratio closer to one to one. While originally thought to be rare, recent epidemiological studies have found lifetime rates of 6.2 percent in psychiatric outpatients and 4–5 percent[4] in community populations. Grant et al. found that of 102 adolescents admitted to a psychiatric inpatient facility, thirteen

(12.7 percent) had a current diagnosis of IED.[5] IED generally appears in adolescence through the twenties and usually runs a course of about twenty years.

There is much comorbidity in individuals with IED with mood, anxiety, substance use, eating, and other impulse control disorders ranging in frequency from 7–89 percent. IED appears to be a separate disorder since it usually has an earlier onset. Although a manic episode may serve as an explanation of an aggressive outburst, there is also a significant amount of overlap of IED with bipolar illness, which may be separate entities or on a continuum of symptoms of irritability, increased energy, and racing thoughts. This comorbidity will be important in treatment with a mood-stabilizing medication being the first line of treatment.[6]

Proposed psychodynamic explanations of impulsive aggression include being a defense against narcissistic injuries with rage outbursts serving to maintain interpersonal distance while psychosocial theories regarding the effect of childhood abuse and neglect deserve consideration in the individual patient who presents for treatment. However, most efforts now concentrate on biological explanations in the hope of developing effective treatments. Genetic and family studies have found higher than expected rates of impulse-control disorders, depressive disorders, and substance use in first degree relatives of individuals with IEDs in addition to increased histories of temper or explosive outbursts.[7] Molecular genetic studies of two populations, 350 Finnish sibling pairs and 305 Southwestern American Indian sibling pairs, found the rate of IED in relatives of antisocial probands to be 15 percent, whereas the relatives of healthy subjects had neither IED nor antisocial personality disorder. It appears that the gene predisposing to antisocial personality and alcoholism lies close to the gene coding for the 5-HT_{1B} serotonin receptor, implicated in impulsivity and aggression.[8]

Biological explanations for aggression, violence, and self-injurious behavior have focused on the brain's prefrontal and anterior cingulate cortex, which tend to be inhibitory, and the limbic regions, including the amygdala and insula, which tend to be excitatory, and particularly on serotonergic neurons within their connecting pathways. Evidence indicates that serotonin- releasing neurons mediate behavioral inhibition and that low levels of serotonin predispose to aggression and decrease the effect of punishment as a deterrent to such behavior. This has been shown by animal studies that diminish the synthesis of serotonin or antagonize its effect while other studies that increase serotonin, by administering precursors or drugs that increase synaptic levels, will restore behavioral effects of punishment and restore control of episodic violence. In humans, low levels of CSF 5-HIAA (a metabolite of serotonin) have been correlated with impulsive aggression while drugs such as selective serotonin reuptake inhibitors (SSRIs), which increase serotonin levels, have decreased the irritability that leads to some episodes of aggression.[9] PET scanning comparing aggressive individuals with controls has demonstrated decreased serotonergic innervation in the anterior cingulate cortex, a region important in affective regulation.[10]

Siever has reviewed the neurobiology of aggression and violence and also includes abnormalities of norepinephrine and dopamine systems in addition to imbalances of the glutamate and GABA systems as contributing to increased aggression. He describes aggression as due to insufficient prefrontal inhibition of limbic-mediated affective responses to stimuli, which produce anger and provoke violent behaviors.[11]

Treatment studies are rare and no drug is specifically approved by the FDA for treatment of IED, but given the evidence regarding the pathological mechanisms, several medications have been tried and found useful. The selective serotonin reuptake inhibitors (SSRIs) that increase serotonin have been helpful while antidepressants that have noradrenergic effects such as the older tricyclics may worsen impulsivity and aggression, which also suggests avoiding the newer dual-action (SNRIs) antidepressants.[12] A recent fourteen-week randomized, double-blind study of fluoxetine in 100 subjects found reduced impulsive aggression compared to baseline but only 44 percent of the fluoxetine responders achieved full remission.[13] The mood stabilizers such as lithium and the anticonvulsants, including carbamazepine and divalproex may decrease neuronal excitability and therefore decrease irritability and impulsivity.[14] Various antipsychotics such as haloperidol, trifluoperazine, and olanzapine have been studied in patients with aggression and borderline personality and findings indicate decrease in anger and hostility, but not depression and other debilitating symptoms. Opiate antagonists may decrease self-injurious behaviors and some of the substance abuse common in aggressive individuals.[15] Benzodiazepines should be avoided as they can decrease inhibition leading to increased loss of control and aggression. Psychotherapy that focuses on anger management and aggression has been tried in these individuals. Cognitive behavioral therapy (CBT) has been studied with results of decreased aggression and anger in the treatment group.[16]

Kleptomania

Individuals with kleptomania fail to resist the urge to steal objects that are not needed for personal use or for monetary value. These individuals rarely use the objects and usually can afford to buy them. As in other impulse control disorders, they describe a sense of rising internal tension that is relieved by the act of stealing. They may later feel guilt or remorse and shame and depression. These individuals are unlikely to steal when immediate arrest is likely and they may not consider the possibility of apprehension, often presenting after being ordered into treatment after repeated arrests.[17, 18] Stealing may also occur from homes of friends and relatives and other nonretail locations.

According to a national survey of 43,000 adults conducted from 2001–2002, 11.3 percent admitted to shoplifting in their lifetime.[19] All antisocial behaviors were strongly associated with shoplifting and 89 percent of the shoplifters had a lifetime psychiatric diagnosis compared to 49.5 percent of the nonshoplifters, while 37 percent of the shoplifters had been treated for mental health problems. While two thirds of the shoplifting occurred before age fifteen, over a third of individuals continued shoplifting after that age, representing 4 percent of the adult population. Kleptomania was not assessed for in this study, but it is likely that some of those who sought mental health treatment were likely to fit the criteria. Grant and colleagues found 8.8 percent of 102 adolescent psychiatric inpatients met current criteria for kleptomania[20] as did sixteen (7.8 percent) of 204 adult inpatients.[21] Meanwhile, a college sample of 791 students found only three (0.38 percent) admitted to symptoms of kleptomania on a self-administered assessment instrument[22]—compatible with the idea that there are two peaks in kleptomania, early adolescence and adulthood around age thirty. Most studies show that there are more females with kleptomania than males, but this may be due to males being sent to correctional settings rather than mental health facilities.[23]

A sample of ninety-five recruited adults who met the criteria for kleptomania was characterized by several instruments.[24] The sample consisted of twenty-seven males and sixty-eight females with a mean age of onset of shoplifting at eighteen years and seven months and a range of onset between six and sixty-two years of age. Two-thirds had been arrested and one-third had served jail or prison time. Men tended to be significantly younger at age of onset of shoplifting and were more likely to steal from electronic goods stores, while women were more likely to steal from stores that sold household goods. Primary triggers for stealing were stress and seeing desired items.

Those suffering from kleptomania commonly also suffer from mood disorders, anxiety disorders, bulimia nervosa, and personality disorders, all of which may bring the person into treatment.[25] Baylé and colleagues found that when compared to a group of sixty patients with alcohol abuse or dependence and twenty-nine psychiatric comparison subjects, eleven patients with kleptomania had higher scores on impulsivity and eight (73 percent) had a lifetime prevalence of a mood disorder.[26] In addition to high frequency of mood disorders, many have other impulse control disorders with 52 percent of men and 26.5 percent of women in the above study of ninety-five adults.[27]

Kleptomania may be related to some brain damage and has been seen in mental retardation and after traumatic injuries.[28] One study looked at neuropsychological functioning of fifteen women with kleptomania and while there was little significant deviation from normal, five subjects did show some impairment in executive functioning.[29] As described in other ICDs, it may be postulated that there is dysfunction in orbitofrontal-subcortical circuits. Grant compared ten females with kleptomania to ten controls by diffusion tensor imaging, an MRI technique measuring the self-diffusion of water in brain tissue, and found compromised white matter integrity in inferior frontal regions.[30] There is little other data regarding the pathophysiology of kleptomania but as in other impulsive disorders, there is the likelihood of a disturbance of monoamine neurotransmitters such as serotonin, while there are similarities to addiction and the reward systems of dopamine and opioid neurotransmission.

Psychoanalytic writers stress the expression of aggressive impulses while others see a libidinal aspect. Some relate the stealing to childhood trauma and abuse or neglect and have conceptualized it as a form of acting out.[31] Kleptomania may fit into the self-medication hypothesis of shoplifting in that the act is an attempt to relieve depressive feelings and low self-esteem.[32]

Due to the low frequency of diagnosis of kleptomania, there have been few clinical trials of treatment options. Co-occurring psychiatric illnesses must be addressed and treated either with some form of psychotherapy or psychopharmacology or both. Insight-oriented psychotherapy may help with the feelings of guilt and shame and uncover some of the underlying motives to steal.[33] Behavior therapies such as systematic desensitization and aversive conditioning have been successful.[34, 35] More recently, cognitive behavior therapy has been used successfully in the related disorder of compulsive shopping and may serve as a model for treatment of kleptomania.[36] The serotonin reuptake inhibitors have shown limited success as have mood stabilizers and other antidepressants and are recently reviewed by Koran et al.[37] and Schreiber et al.[38] Grant has published several studies on successful treatment with the opioid antagonist naltrexone, supporting the relationship between this impulse control disorder and the reward system.[39] A recent case report by Talih describes an integrated treatment approach in a patient with kleptomania.[40]

Pyromania

Pyromania is characterized by multiple episodes of deliberate fire setting, feelings of tension or affective arousal prior to setting a fire, fascination and attraction to fires, and experiences of pleasure or relief of tension after setting the fire. Additionally, the fire setting is not done for financial gain, to conceal criminal activity, to express anger or vengeance, or done in response to a delusion. The fire setting cannot result from the impaired judgment of dementia, mental retardation, intoxication, or in the context of a diagnosis of conduct disorder, manic episode, or antisocial personality.[41] Individuals with pyromania may spend a lot of time preparing for starting a fire, are fascinated by fire, and may spend a significant amount of time watching fires. They may set off fire alarms and may be indifferent to the consequences or may even get satisfaction from the destruction resulting from the fire.[42]

Pyromania itself is thought to be relatively rare since most cases of fire setting and arson are the result of actions by individuals meeting the criteria for antisocial personality, conduct disorder, and substance intoxication, which are exclusionary criteria for pyromania.[43, 44] Juvenile fire setting is common, and it is estimated that 60 percent of all fires are set by those between eleven and eighteen years of age with males more common than females. Epidemiological studies have demonstrated the prevalence of fire setting to be between 2.4–3.5 percent in this age group.[45] A prevalence study on fire setting by adults in the US by National Epidemiologic Survey on Alcohol and Related Conditions (NESARC) found that 1.13 percent of the surveyed population acknowledged fire setting over their lifetime with most of those individuals also meeting criteria for antisocial personality, drug dependence, bipolar disorder, or pathological gambling.[46] However, three recent studies by Grant and colleagues identified a prevalence of 1 percent in a college sample,[47] and a lifetime prevalence of 5.9 percent in adult psychiatric inpatients,[48] while 6.9 percent of an adolescent inpatient psychiatric population met the criteria for pyromania.[49]

Psychological explanations for pyromania include Freud's belief that fire was a symbol of sexuality, while other analysts associated pyromania with a craving for power and prestige. Some pyromaniacs have volunteered as firefighters or have tried to prove themselves as brave by putting out the blaze.[50] Grant and Kim were able to recruit twenty-one adult and adolescent subjects with pyromania and described high levels of comorbid mood disorders (62 percent), and other impulse control disorders (47.6 percent), suggesting a similar underlying neuropathology for multiple behaviors characterized by reward-seeking.[51] Substance abuse and anxiety disorders were also common, with 33 percent lifetime prevalence for each. As in other impulsive disorders, low levels of serotonin and norepinephrine have been suggested due to low levels of their metabolites in the CSF of fire setters.[52] A recent case report of an eighteen-year old male with pyromania described a SPECT (Single Photon Emission Computed Tomography) scan that revealed a left inferior frontal perfusion deficit that resolved after twelve months of treatment, which included cognitive behavioral therapy and topiramate.[53]

Treatment approaches to pyromania have been similar to other impulse control disorders and include behavior therapy with aversive conditioning, positive reinforcement, and social skills training.[54, 55] Pyromania that co-occurs with mood disorders or substance abuse problems should be treated appropriately with mood stabilizers like topiramate[56] or SSRIs, such as escitalopram, sertraline, and fluoxetine[57] or antipsychotics for psychotic symptoms.

Trichotillomania

Recurrent hair pulling is the main symptom of trichotillomania. *DSM-IV-TR* lists five criteria for trichotillomania: The sufferer pulls out enough hair that hair loss is noticeable, most commonly from the scalp, but can also affect axillary areas, pubic hair, eyebrows, and eyelashes (Criteria A). Hair pulling can occur in response to stressful times, but can also occur during relaxation such as while reading a book. Also, about 75 percent of adults report that their hair pulling is automatic or outside their awareness, while the other 25 percent say they are focused on the behavior while engaging in it. The individual feels increasing tension prior to the act or from the attempt to resist the urge. (Criteria B) There is a feeling of gratification, pleasure, or sense of relief following the hair pulling. (Criteria C) Criteria B and C are controversial since some individuals who pull out hair do not report, or recognize, these feelings.[58]

Trichotillomania is not diagnosed if the hair pulling is due to another condition such as delusions or hallucinations or a medical condition such as inflammation of the skin. (Criteria D) And, the condition must cause significant distress or impairment in important areas of functioning such as social and occupational (Criteria E).

Trichotillomania was first described in 1889 by the French dermatologist François Hallopeau. It is more common in women than men, frequent in children where it peaks at ages twelve to thirteen, and occurs in about 1.5 percent of males and 3.4

percent of females.[59] Hair pullers may also eat the hair, called trichophagia, which may lead to trichobezoars and intestinal obstruction. Grant and Odlaug found that fourteen of sixty-eight individuals with trichotillomania were current hair eaters and more likely to be male than in the total population of hair-pullers.[60] Sufferers frequently have comorbid mood disorders, anxiety disorders, substance abuse problems, personality disorders, and mental retardation.[61, 62] There is some thought that trichotillomania should be classified as a variant of OCD due to the repetitive and uncontrollable nature of hair pulling; however, the behavior is not accompanied by the unwanted intrusive thoughts of OCD.[63]

Some theories link hair pulling to stressful situations, including disturbances in the mother-child relationship, fear of being left alone, and recent object loss. Genetic influences are important with family members having histories of tics, impulse control disorders, and obsessive-compulsive symptoms. As in other impulse control disorders, abnormalities in the serotonin and opioid systems are suspected of playing a role. Recent reviews of trichotillomania discuss neuroimaging and cognitive function extensively.[64, 65] Some neuroimaging studies have demonstrated decreases in volume compared to normal in the frontal regions, the putamen, and the cerebellum but these studies are sometimes contradicted by other studies.[66] When cognitive function has been evaluated in hair pullers, problems in visuospatial learning and response inhibition have been identified. Since response inhibition is affected by the norepinephrine system, the system also most associated with anxiety and feelings of tension, dysregulation of this system might serve as an explanation for the pathophysiology of trichotillomania.

Treatment studies are few but tend to support a combination of behavioral and medication therapies. Habit reversal, a behavioral therapy with a long history for treatment of nervous habits, aims to substitute a competing, harmless motor response to the urge to pull hair. Two studies showed improvement although benefits were diminished at long-term follow-up.[67] A letter from Trainor described success with CBT in treating children with trichotillomania.[68] While several trials of various medications have been done, most studies consisted of small sample size and showed little efficacy.[69] Clomipramine showed slight superiority over desipramine, but the lack of a placebo limited the study. Fluoxetine, an SSRI, did not show an advantage over placebo in two studies, while a study of naltrexone, an opioid antagonist, did show some improvement compared to placebo. Another study looked at the antipsychotic olanzapine, and those with trichotillomania did better than those on placebo, supporting the idea that it is similar to motor tics.[70] One recent study by Grant found that N-acetylcysteine, an amino acid found in health food stores that modulates glutamate in the CNS, reduced frequency of hair pulling and improved overall feelings in just over half of the participants.[71]

Two studies comparing CBT to medication found that CBT was superior to clomipramine and placebo in a study with a small number of participants, while a similar study found behavior therapy superior to fluoxetine and a wait-list group. Therefore, it is suggested that medication be reserved for severe cases or those with comorbid illnesses where the medication is a first-line drug and that the focus of treatment be on the behavior itself and the social conditions that are contributing to the unwanted behavior.[72] Grant and colleagues' recent book, *Trichotillomania, Skin Picking, and Other Body-Focused Repetitive Behaviors*, describes several treatments, particularly psychotherapies, of trichotillomania in extensive detail.

Impulse Control Disorder Not Otherwise Specified

DSM-IV-TR includes this residual diagnostic category for disorders of impulse control that do not meet the criteria for a specific impulse control disorder. It has been proposed that sexual compulsive behavior, problematic Internet usage, compulsive shopping, and self-injurious behavior belong in this group,[73,][74] with the first two of these problems discussed in Chapters Four and Seven of this book. Sadock and Sadock discuss the subtle distinction between impulse and compulsion, with an impulse being a tension state that can exist without an action while a compulsion always includes an action component.[75] Also, impulses are acted on with the expectation of a feeling of pleasure or relief while compulsions are generally unpleasant and undesired. *DSM-5,* as of this writing, proposes to move several of the disorders of impulse control into new groupings as discussed below.

Impulse Control Disorders and Substance Use Disorders

There are several similarities between substance use disorders and some of the impulse control disorders, particularly pathological gambling, kleptomania, compulsive shopping, and compulsive Internet use. The behaviors share common features with the core elements of addiction, including an urge to engage in a behavior with negative consequences, mounting tension until the behavior is completed, rapid but temporary resolution of the urge following the action, return of the urge, external cues unique to the behavior, secondary conditioning by internal and external cues such as boredom and dysphoria, and a hedonic feeling early in the addiction.[76] The impulse behaviors have a pleasurable quality and the individual may spend time contemplating and planning the behavior in spite of the possibility of negative consequences. Additionally, performance of the action may result in diminished anxiety or dysphoria as does the use of most addictive substances.

Evidence linking the impulse control disorders with substance addictions includes the genetic studies where there is a higher frequency of substance use disorders in relatives of individuals with impulse control disorders, in addition to those with ICDs having higher incidences of substance use problems. Also, the same neurotransmitters and neurocircuits are implicated in both sets of disorders while promising treatment studies with drugs, such as the opioid antagonists, again suggest a strong relation.[77] One of the most intriguing questions is why a specific behavior or drug is "chosen" to relieve the tension or as Hollander suggests that a different motivational salience alters the functional neurocircuitry for each disorder. He gives the examples that pathologic gamblers' behavior is in response to the potential monetary reward, in the same way binge eaters respond to food and those who are sexually compulsive respond to sexual stimuli.[78] It will be important to consider the environment in which individuals are raised to assess what activities were available, encouraged, discouraged, rewarded, or punished in understanding some of the learning aspects of these disorders.

DSM-5

DSM-5 is expected to be published in May of 2013. The Impulse Control Disorders will undergo some changes in the proposed manual as it now stands. Trichotillomania, to be known as Hair-Pulling Disorder, will move into the Obsessive-Compulsive and Related Disorders category and will be joined by its related diagnosis of Skin Picking Disorder. Impulse Control Disorders Not Elsewhere Classified will join with Disorders Usually First Diagnosed in Infancy, Childhood, or Adolescence into a new category called Disruptive, Impulse Control, and Conduct Disorders. Pyromania, Kleptomania, and Intermittent Explosive Disorder will remain together in this category with the criteria for Intermittent Explosive Disorder presently being finalized. Pathological gambling is being renamed Gambling Disorder and will move into the Substance Use and Addictive Disorders category.[79]

7

Internet Addiction

An-Pyng Sun, PhD, LCSW

Historical Background

Although the Internet and computers contribute exponentially to the technological and cultural advancement of humankind, it is not an overstatement to say that the negative consequences of their misuse among some people can be equivalent to those of the most addictive legal or illegal drugs such as alcohol and heroin. "Internet addiction" has, in the past two decades, caused a great deal of concern from society in general and clinicians in particular because of the problems and negative implications related to it.

This phenomenon has been noticed in many countries around the globe, including those in North America, Asia, and Europe. The problem of Internet addiction is especially prevalent in some Asian countries, such as China, South Korea, and Taiwan. The perception of the severity of this epidemic by society in China and Taiwan has propelled a new term— "electronic opium" or "digital dope"—to label the addictive

Internet games and activities, and a new term—"the New Opium War"—to represent the war combating this problem, in reference to the nineteenth century Opium War occurring between China and Great Britain. Some astounding actual cases reported in the media related to Internet addiction in recent years include: addicts who died of cardiac arrest due to the uncontrollable binge use of Internet games and a subsequent deprivation of sleep and food; addicts who starved their infants to death because of their prolonged immersion in the virtual world; and addicts who attacked or even killed their parents because of the parents' attempts to stop them from engaging in computer games.

In 2007, a seventeen-year-old Ohio teenage boy shot and killed his mother and injured his father because they took away his computer video game. The boy was sentenced to twenty-three years in prison. The judge said that the boy's obsession with the video game may have led him to believe that "death wasn't real," just like those creatures in the game.

Also in 2007, the *Associated Press* reported that a thirty-year-old man lost his life to an Internet gaming binge. This man suffered from depletion after playing the game for three days in a row in a southern China city. Paramedics tried to revive him but failed. The article went on to say that he may have died from exhaustion brought on by too many hours on the Internet.

In 2012, another young Chinese/Taiwanese man died of binge use of Internet games. This happened in New Taipei City, Taiwan. According to the *Formosa News*, the twenty-three-year-old man died after a twenty-three-hour binge of Internet games. His body was stiff, with one hand still on the keyboard and the other on the mouse, when the police found him. The doctor said the death could be related to a cardiac arrest, due to problematic blood circulation and the cold weather. The Internet café owner said that the young man was a regular customer who came to the café three or four days a week, reserving a station for at least eight hours each time when he was there.

Although Internet addiction has caught the attention of many clinicians in the field, as well as society in general, the *DSM-5* work group has been cautious regarding whether or not to add this new pathology to the updated *DSM* and place it under a formal diagnostic category. At this time, the *DSM-5* work group has recommended including "Internet Addiction" in its appendix (Section Three) to stimulate more research on this issue, instead of placing it in the newly proposed category of "Substance Use and Other Addictive Disorders," which includes substance use disorder and gambling disorder. The *DSM-5* work group presently determines that more research is needed to confirm the status of "Internet Addiction" as a formal psychiatric diagnosis.

The concept of Internet addiction is controversial and experts debate whether the addiction exists in and of itself, for at least four reasons. First is the concern of possibly too low a threshold. The perspective is that if every satisfied urge or desire, for example from an illicit drug to fashionable handbags, can be considered as a symptom manifested from addiction, the term "addiction" will explain everything but then also virtually nothing.[1] Petry holds the same view, stating that ". . . as we move forward in understanding more clearly how, why, and who engages in problematic Internet gaming, we should also consider the past. The Internet gaming 'addiction' of the early twenty-first century may be reminiscent of video arcade and television 'addiction' from the previous generation. If we draw the threshold too low, all excessive behavior patterns, including eating too much chocolate and working too much, may become psychiatric disorders . . . ."[2] She believes that more data need to be collected regarding the how, why, and who of addiction to Internet games and activities before we classify Internet addiction as a psychiatric disorder, and that if we adopt too low of a threshold, we may eventually limit treatment coverage for clients who have real psychiatric disorders. To differentiate between features of addiction and characteristics of new lifestyles is challenging.[3]

The second concern is the possibility of over-prescribing. This concern was voiced by psychiatrist Allen Frances, the chair of the 1994 *DSM-IV* task force. Dr. Frances considers many of the *DSM-5* proposed revisions to be negative changes, which may result in over-prescribing. He said that the *DSM-5* task force members are completely naïve concerning how the contents in the book are converted in the real world.[4]

The third reason some scholars and practitioners hesitate to consider Internet addiction as a formal psychiatric disorder is that they are uncertain whether Internet addiction is in and of itself a discrete disease, rather than secondary to a primary diagnosis. In other words, they worry that the concept of "Internet addiction" may be erroneous and may in fact, be a manifestation of symptoms of other underlying primary psychiatric diagnoses, such as bipolar disorder, major depressive disorder, anxiety disorder, and so on.[5] This issue is highlighted especially since problematic Internet use often appears in the context of co-occurring disorders.

One last reason for doubt about Internet addiction as a discrete disorder is that some experts believe that many studies involved with the topic are flawed methodologically.[6]

There are responses to the above concerns that delay the classification of "Internet addiction" to be a formal psychiatric disorder. For example, one of the strongest supporters of categorizing Internet addiction as a psychiatric disorder is Elias Aboujaoude, who wrote, "Simply stating that similar fears have been raised with every new technology misses the point: The immersive and interactive qualities of the virtual medium, combined with its sheer penetration into every aspect of life, make it different from all media forms that preceded it . . . ."[7] In addition, although Shapira et al. consider that more research is necessary to determine Internet addiction to be a discrete disease entity, they also agree that some evidence exists suggesting that not all problematic Internet use can be explained by other conditions and that similar to other impulse control disorders, it can be prevalent and disabling.[8] Although Pies does not think we have enough evidence yet to label

Internet addiction a distinct disease entity, he does believe that more and more research indicates that professional treatment is needed by some individuals who are afflicted with Internet addiction.[9] Shaw and Black suggest that we should not ignore Internet addiction, because if we do, it would only stigmatize and trivialize our attempts to understand it better and treat it.[10]

Regardless of whether Internet addiction exists and whether it qualifies for a designation of a formal psychiatric diagnosis under *DSM-5*, in recent years we have seen tragic stories and cases related to Internet obsession and misuse—from the media and addiction treatment programs in the United States as well as internationally. Such tragedies have often implicated not only the addicted persons themselves, but also their parents and children. Practitioners in many countries, ranging from China and South Korea to Germany, France, and Greece, and here in the United States, have encountered clients who are afflicted with uncontrollable Internet use and its implications.

Learning how to identify a client with Internet addiction risk early and provide effective assessment and treatment for the client and his or her family are important. The purpose of this chapter is to introduce the knowledge we have so far regarding this epidemic. Types and prevalence rates of Internet addiction, as well as screening, assessment, and treatment strategies are discussed.

Types of Internet Addiction

"Internet addiction" is an umbrella term that can involve various forms and activities and includes at least six different types: 1) computer and online video game addiction, such as being addicted to the massive multiplayer online role playing games; 2) information overload, such as web-surfing addiction; 3) online gambling; 4) online shopping; 5) cybersexual addiction, such as online pornography; and 6) cyber-relationship addiction (e.g., addicted to social networking sites).[11] Young describes two types of Internet addicts. The Classic Addicts are those with a prior history of sex, gambling, or substance addiction who found the

Internet to be a new or safer outlet to fulfill their addictions. The New Addicts are individuals without a history of prior addiction whose addiction to the Internet is completely a new problem.[12]

Prevalence Rates

Prevalence rates of Internet addiction may be somewhat inconsistent for various reasons, including their existence in different regions and countries whose rates may be affected by different cultural and social factors; adopting different measurement tools; surveying different populations or subpopulations that contain different distributions of age and gender groups; and using different research designs and sampling methods. Studies may adopt different measuring tools to determine whether an individual is positive or negative with respect to Internet addiction. For example, some used Young's Internet Addiction Test scale, whereas others used Young's Diagnostic Questionnaire or Morahan-Martin and Schumacher's Pathological Internet Use Scale.[13]

Some tools separate the screening or assessment outcomes into nonaddicted, moderately addicted, and severely addicted; whereas others differentiate the results only into addicted or not addicted. Whether or not "moderately addicted" and the "maladaptive Internet use" should be counted as addiction further creates confusion and inconsistency among the various reported prevalence rates. Some studies are general population-based, whereas others focus on universities and high schools or other specific subpopulations. Likewise, some studies treat Internet addiction as an umbrella term and investigate the issue in an inclusive manner, whereas others target only computer/Internet gaming, for example. Furthermore, some use probability sampling methods, many others, however, use nonprobability sampling methods.

Two population-based cross-sectional studies have been done and prevalence rates varied from 0.7 percent from a study of the United States to 1.0 percent in Norway. These two rates are not too far apart despite their representing different countries and using different measuring tools. Aboujaoude et al. conducted an epidemiological study (N = 2,513; mean age = 48.5; 68.89 percent of the 2,513 adults were regular Internet users) of problematic Internet use using a random-digit-dial telephone survey in the United States.[14] They defined problematic Internet use using four different sets of criteria; the first set was the least restrictive and included three conditions: a) the individual's relationships are interfered with by Internet use; b) the individual is preoccupied with the Internet when offline; and c) the individual has "either tried unsuccessfully to cut down on Internet use or stayed online longer than intended 'often' or 'very often.'"[15] The results, based on this least restrictive set of criteria, showed that 0.7 percent of the total population surveyed met the criteria for problematic Internet use disorder. The rate of 0.7 percent may not completely represent today's situation because the study was conducted in 2004 and the percentage of regular users then was only 69 percent, which could have increased today.

Using a stratified probability sampling method, Bakken and colleagues studied 3,399 Norwegians aged sixteen through seventy-four (87.1 percent of the 3,399 were Internet users). They used Young's Diagnostic Questionnaire, which includes eight yes/no questions and considers an individual Internet addicted if he or she answered with yes five or more times. Their results showed that 1.0 percent of the population met the five or more criteria and thus were classified as Internet addicted; 5.2 percent of the population met three to four criteria and were considered as at-risk Internet users.[16]

In addition to general population-based studies, many other studies targeted school or university students or other subpopulations, using probability or nonprobability sampling methods. The prevalence rates of Internet addiction or problematic Internet use usually ranged from 6 to 23 percent, which are considerably higher than those from the general population-based studies. The US nongeneral population studies showed rates of 8 to 9 percent.

Morahan-Martin and Schumacher studied 277 US undergraduates who were Internet users, using the Pathological Internet Use Scale (PIU). The results showed about 27.2 percent reporting no symptoms; 64.7 percent reporting limited symptoms (meeting one to three of the thirteen conditions related to withdrawal symptoms, mood-altering use, personal distress, work problems, academic problems, or interpersonal problems, etc.); and 8.1 percent, reporting pathological Internet use (meeting four or more of the thirteen conditions).[17] Gentile's 2009 study (US youths aged eight to eighteen) showed a similar rate of 8.5 percent, despite his concentrating only on the video-game players (versus Internet use in general) and using a different measuring tool. Gentile defined pathological patterns of play as exhibiting six or more of eleven symptoms of impairment related to family, social, school, or psychological functioning. Gentile stated that although the rate of 8.5 percent may seem high, it is similar to the pathological video-game use rates in other studies with a similar age group, such as 9.9 percent among Spanish teenagers.[18]

The non-US, nongeneral population studies, mostly on adolescent and young adults, showed rates between 6 to 23 percent. Again, the vast gap among the rates could be attributable to the usage of different definitions and measurement tools for Internet addiction, as well as different research designs, including probability versus nonprobability sampling methods. Some studies targeting adolescents and young adults in China indicated prevalence rates of about 2.4 to 11 percent; a German study found 12 percent; a South Korean study showed 10.7 percent; a study done in Taiwan indicated 23.4 percent; and a Greek study reported 20.9 percent maladaptive Internet use. A Lebanon study indicated 4.2 percent.

Based on Young's Internet Addiction Test (IAT), a study in Guangzhou City, China, (N = 1,618 high school students, aged thirteen to eighteen) found that about 89.2 percent of the respondents were normal users (scores between twenty and forty-nine); 10.2 percent were moderately addicted (scores between fifty and seventy-nine); and 0.6 percent were severely addicted (scores between eighty and one hundred).[19] Also using Young's IAT, but dividing the outcomes into four groups instead of three, Hawi's 2012 study with web-based questionnaires, (N = 833 intermediate and secondary students in Lebanon) showed that 21.8 percent scored less than twenty points (not addicted); 39.2 percent, twenty to thirty-nine points ("has complete control over his or her usage"); 34.9 percent, forty to sixty-nine points ("frequent problems due to Internet usage"); and 4.2 percent, seventy to one hundred points ("the Internet is causing significant problems").[20]

Also adopting Young's IAT, Park, Kim, and Cho's 2009 study (N = 903) of middle and high school students in Seoul, South Korea found that 10.7 percent of the respondents met the Internet addiction criteria; 73.7 percent possible Internet addiction; and 15.0 percent no addiction.[21] In China, Ni, Yan, Chen, and Liu's 2009 study (N = 3,557 freshmen university students) found that 6.44 percent of the respondents met the criteria for Internet addiction with a Young IAT score greater than fifty.[22] A German study (7,069 gamers; 94 percent male; mean age = 21.11 years, SD = 6.35), in collaborating with an online gaming magazine to recruit participants and by using the six criteria of addiction established by the World Health Organization's ICD-10, found that 11.9 percent of the respondents met three or more of the six criteria and thus were considered as pathological gamers.[23] A study of senior high school students in Taiwan (N = 1,289) revealed that 23.4 percent of the respondents met at least five of the eight criteria of the Young's Diagnostic Questionnaire and thus were classified as addicted Internet users.[24] A Greek study (N = 866 randomly selected adolescents; mean age = 14.7 years) showed that 20.9 percent of the respondents met the criteria of overall maladaptive Internet use, including 19.4 percent potential problematic Internet use and 1.5 percent problematic Internet use, according to Young's Internet Addiction Test.[25]

Risk Factors

Most studies that investigate risk factors for Internet addiction are cross-sectional, not prospective; the nature of the risk factors, therefore, tends to be correlational and the risk factors do not necessarily represent the causes of Internet addiction. The risk factors could be precursors or consequences, or simply factors related to something to which the Internet addiction happens to also be related.

Gender

Out of nineteen studies reviewed, ten indicated that men are more at risk than women for Internet addiction;[26] seven showed no significant difference between men and women;[27] and two suggested that women are more likely than men to be addicted to the Internet.[28, 29]

One explanation for the gender difference could be that males are more likely than females to engage in cybersex, online gambling, and online gaming, all of which tend to be more addictive than other types of Internet activities.[30, 31] For example, Hawi's 2012 study indicates that among the various Internet activities, more women than men prefer communication and messaging (86.7 percent versus 78.1 percent, respectively), and more men than women prefer entertainment, e.g., gaming (63.2 percent versus 42.1 percent, respectively).[32] The two studies that found women are more likely than men to be addicted to the Internet (i.e., Young, 1998 and Andreassen, 2012) both focused only on the area of online communication or Facebook.

Reward Deficiency Syndrome

Internet or other manifestations of addiction may be related to an individual's abnormal brain reward cascade. Research has suggested that the main loci for an individual's feelings of reward and well-being are in the individual's mesolimbic dopaminergic centers, and some individuals—especially those with a family history of addiction—may be born with a deficiency of dopamine receptors and function, resulting in a lack of usual feelings of satisfaction and an ability to cope with pressure.[33] The reward deficiency syndrome may also be acquired through prolonged exposure to stress and alcohol or other drugs. An individual with predisposed or acquired reward deficiency syndrome may pursue psychoactive substances (such as alcohol, amphetamines, cannabinoids, opiates), and/ or indulge in thrill-seeking behaviors (such as sex, gambling, overeating, video gaming) to overcome the anhedonic condition by stimulating the mesolimbic dopaminergic centers.[34]

In 2009, Ko and colleagues compared ten respondents with online gaming addiction and ten respondents without such an addiction (the control group). They found that several regions of the brain (right orbitofrontal cortex, bilateral anterior cingulate, medial frontal cortex, right nucleus accumbens, right dorsolateral prefrontal cortex, and right caudate nucleus) were activated when the addicted respondent viewed the gaming-related pictures, whereas such activation did not occur when the addicted respondent viewed the mosaic pictures or when the control respondent viewed the gaming-related pictures.[35] The activation of those brain areas was also positively related to the respondent's self-reported gaming urge. Ko et al.'s study further demonstrated that the regions of the brain that were activated in the cue-induced craving in online gaming addiction are similar to those in substance dependence.

Low Emotional Well-Being

Emotional well-being may include indicators such as levels of self-esteem, stress, loneliness, social support, and so on. One issue here is that it is uncertain whether these indicators and symptoms are precursors or consequences or both with respect to Internet addiction. For example, loneliness could lead to Internet addiction, which functions to compensate for a person's isolation, boredom, and inadequate interpersonal relationships in the real world. However, Internet addiction could also result in loneliness; a person's indulgence in the virtual world may alienate his or her interactions with people in the real world.

Many studies found the coexistence of problematic Internet use or stress to be a predictor of Internet addiction. Lam and colleagues' logistic regression analyses show that a young person's experiencing "recent stressful events" may be related to Internet addiction.[36] A person with high stress related to a recent event was ten times more likely, and a person with moderate stress related to a recent event was 2.8 times more likely than a person with no recent stressful event or experiencing no stress despite stressful events to be at risk for Internet addiction.[37] Controlling for age, gender, and amount of time weekly playing video-games, Gentile found a linkage between pathological Internet use and poorer school performance.[38] Wang et al. reported an association between problematic Internet use and factors of impoverished classmate relationships and study-related stress among students.[39] Wang et al. suggested that the Internet may provide a refuge for adolescents to escape from reality, as well as to seek acceptance.[40] Li, Wang, and Wang's 2009 study found that problematic Internet use was related not only to stress, but also to an individual's coping style.[41] Specifically, the problematic use group experienced a significantly higher number of stressful events in the past half-year than the nonproblematic use group; the problematic use group also used more avoidant coping and less problem-solving strategies than the nonproblematic use group. Li et al. suggest that stressful life events may serve as a preexisting mechanism of problematic Internet use and such problematic use is mediated by avoidant coping style, which includes withdrawal, rationalization, self-blame, and fantasy.[42]

Loneliness may be a risk factor for Internet addiction. Morahan-Martin and Schumacher said that individuals who are socially or emotionally isolated may engage in Internet use, which often offers more attractive or exciting substitutes for an unhappy or ordinary life.[43] Using the UCLA Loneliness

Scale, Morahan-Martin and Schumacher (277 undergraduate Internet users, US) found that problematic users had a significantly higher loneliness score (M = 46.14, SD = 7.11) than both those with limited symptoms (M = 38.38, SD = 7.79) and those with no symptoms did (M = 35.86, SD = 9.36). These results are similar to Nalwa and Anand's study (100 students aged sixteen to eighteen, India). They found that the Internet dependents had a significantly higher UCLA Loneliness Scale score (M = 47.5; SD = 9.15) than the nondependents (M = 37.7; SD = 11.13).[44]

Ni et al. studied freshmen college students and found that those whose hometowns were not where the university was located were at a higher risk for Internet addiction and infer that they may feel loneliness because of homesickness and being unacquainted with the environment.[45] All three studies are cross-sectional in nature, and it is uncertain whether the factor of loneliness takes place prior to the Internet addiction. The direction of the relationship between Internet addiction and loneliness may be paradoxical. Two longitudinal studies showed contradictory results. Chen, Li, and Long et al. measured 382 undergraduates regarding their levels of social support during the end of first term of their freshmen year and the students were followed afterwards for four and a half years to gather the incidence rate of Internet addiction.[46] Their results showed that those with high social support or perceived social support were less likely to develop Internet addiction; the rates were 2.4 percent, 7.9 percent, and 15.7 percent for the participants whose social support score were greater than 73, 61–73, and 0–60, respectively.

On the other hand, Kraut et al.'s longitudinal study shows that preexisting loneliness does not predict problematic Internet use; rather, problematic Internet use leads to increased loneliness because of decreased social interactions and connections with the real-life world.[47] More prospective studies with sound research designs are needed in this regard.

Psychiatric Disorders

Extensive studies have consistently shown that among adolescents and young adults, Internet addiction is associated with various psychiatric disorders, including affective disorders (e.g., depression), anxiety disorders (generalized anxiety or social anxiety), attention deficit hyperactivity disorder (ADHD), and hostility.[48] However, because of the cross-sectional research designs of many of the studies, a causal relationship between some of these psychiatric diagnoses and the Internet addiction cannot necessarily be inferred. More prospective research with sound designs is needed to establish a causal relationship between the two variables.

Depression is one major psychiatric disorder linked to Internet addiction. Lin et al.'s study (3,616 college students in Taiwan) found that among the various psychosocial risk factors (e.g., positive expectancy of Internet use, hours of Internet usage per week, impulsivity, satisfaction with academic performance, male gender, and insecure attachment style), depressive symptomology is the most influential risk factor for Internet addiction.[49] Yen, Ko, Yen, Chang, and Cheng (N = 8,941, mean age = 14.7, SD = 1.7, Southern Taiwan) found that depression was most powerful in discriminating adolescent Internet addiction.[50] A Korean study also revealed an association between depression and Internet addiction among adolescents.[51] Analyses of the 2007 and 2009 Youth Risk Behavior Survey (YRBS) data (N = 14,041 and N = 16,410, respectively; high school-based representative samples, US) showed a connection between excessive video game/Internet use and teen depression and suicide. The 2009 YRBS data showed that teens who played video games/Internet for five hours or more daily were significantly more likely to report feeling sadness, suicidal ideation (1.7 times more likely), and suicide planning (1.5 times more likely).[52]

Ko et al. attribute the association between Internet addiction and depression to the possibilities that the Internet provides the satisfaction of control, achievement, social support, and a virtual world that allows individuals to avoid emotional difficulties encountered in the real world, all of which appear to alleviate depression and alter mood, but ultimately precipitate a vicious cycle of Internet addiction among vulnerable populations.[53] Citing Wrase and colleagues' study, Ko et al. said the coexistence of Internet addiction and depression could also be because they both are associated with the "short" alleles of the 5HTTLPR gene.[54]

Various studies also show a strong link between ADHD and Internet addiction.[55, 56] Yen et al.'s study indicated that attention deficit, followed by impulsivity, was associated with Internet addiction.[57] Using DuPaul's ADHD rating scale (Korean version; rated by parents and teachers of the students), Yoo et al.'s study of 752 elementary school students found that compared with the nonaddiction group, the Internet addiction group showed a significantly higher score in inattention, hyperactivity-impulsivity, and both combined.[58] Ko et al. stated that individuals with ADHD usually experience "being easily bored" and "having an aversion for delayed reward," both of which may result in worsened academic performance and impaired interpersonal relationships. Internet activities, on the other hand, offer quick responses and reward, as well as various windows of different actions, all of which lessen the sense of boredom and supply immediate stimulation.[59] Ko et al. additionally suggest neurophysiological factors in explaining the coexistence of Internet addiction and ADHD. Citing Koepp et al., Ko et al. stated that when engaging in gaming, the striatal dopamine may be released, which enhances the player's concentration and leads to better performance. Such an effect may help counteract the frustrations these individuals often face in real life.[60] Ko et al. also posed that adolescents with ADHD may have anomalous brain activities related to reduced inhibition, which lowers the adolescents' self-control and leads to their uncontrollable Internet use; or motivation deficit, which promotes a higher level of quick adaptation to repeated positive reinforcement but a lower level of behavioral response or stimulation to punishment.[61]

Family Dysfunction

This risk factor may be more relevant to adolescents, and studies have consistently demonstrated an association between a dysfunctional family and an adolescent's Internet addiction. Those studies are mostly from the Far East, specifically China; very few are from the West. This is perhaps because of the recent dramatic increase of Internet use and Internet addiction among adolescents in Asia, as well as the important role a family assumes in Asian culture. According to those studies, under the umbrella of poor family functioning are ineffective parental monitoring of adolescents' Internet use, high conflicts between the adolescents and family, domestic violence, adolescents' overall dissatisfaction with family, and parental divorce or single-parent family.

On the other hand, family warmth serves as a protective factor. Many empirical studies show consistently that parental supervision and monitoring of Internet usage can inhibit or deter adolescents' Internet addiction.[62, 63] Wang et al.'s study (N = 12,446 high school students who were Internet users, China) indicates that high parent-adolescent conflicts predict adolescents' Internet addiction.[64] Adolescents with conflictive family relations were 2.01 times more likely, and those with very conflictive family relations were 2.60 times more likely to be addicted to the Internet than adolescents with very supportive family relations. Wang et al. stated that high conflicts between adolescents and family contribute to lower adolescent-family involvement, as well as adolescents' refusal to comply with family rules and parental monitoring. Lam, Peng, Mai, and Jing also found that compared with students who were satisfied with their family, those who were very dissatisfied were about approximately 2.5 times more likely to develop an Internet addiction.[65]

Park, Kim, and Cho's study of middle and high school students in Seoul, South Korea (N = 903) indicates that exposure to domestic violence—conjugal or parent-to-child—was associated with adolescents' Internet addiction.[66] Zhang et al.'s logistic regression analysis (N = 4,877 high school students, China) shows that adolescents whose parents were divorced were 1.6 times more likely than other adolescents to be Internet addicted.[67] Likewise, Ni, Yan, Chen, and Liu (3,557 students from a general university in China) also found that having a single-parent family is a risk factor for Internet addiction among adolescents.[68] Finally, Zhang et al.'s study shows that the more an adolescent perceives a warm relationship with his or her parents, the less likely that the adolescent will develop an addiction to the Internet.[69]

The Content Factor

The literature strongly suggests that Internet content preference is a predictor for Internet addiction, especially the sites of sex-related content, gaming, gambling, and chatting. Kormas et al.'s 2011 study shows that compared with adolescent normal Internet users, adolescents with problematic Internet use were 2.7 times more likely to use the Internet to seek sexual information, two times more likely to access the Internet to target interactive game-playing and chat-room, yet significantly less likely to use the Internet to pursue education.[70] Likewise, Ko et al. found a significant relationship between types of Internet activity engaged and later development of Internet addiction.[71] Specifically, the percentages for respondents engaging in online games were 36 percent for the nonaddicted group and 60 percent for the addicted group; in online chatting were 46.2 percent and 36 percent, respectively; and in information search were 17.8 percent and 4 percent, respectively. Wang et al.'s 2011 study further reports that as the level of Internet addiction increased, the interest in using the Internet for information and research activity purpose decreased.[72]

The Time Factor

Available study results revealed at least three themes under the time factor: Internet addiction may be related to age of first Internet use; participants in their earlier phases of engaging in

Internet-related activities may be more likely to have addictive tendencies than their more longer-term and stable counterparts; individuals who spend a greater amount of time in Internet sessions may be more at risk for Internet addiction than the individuals who spend a lesser amount of time.

Zhou, Tang, and Peng's 2009 study found that addicted individuals begin their Internet use at a significantly younger age than nonaddicted individuals.[73] Studies also suggest that newer game players or Internet users—who were perhaps dazzled by their exciting initial encountering experience— may be more likely to show addictive tendencies than their longer-term counterparts who probably had passed the early novelty period and developed more balanced responses to the stimulus.[74] Young's 1998 study indicated that most of the addicted Internet users had been online for less than one year, whereas nonaddicted users tend to be online more than one year.[75] Young thus suggested that the Internet Addiction Test should be used with caution when assessing novice Internet users during their initial half-year of exposure. For novice users, the excessive amount of time devoted to Internet usage may be related to their new and exciting experience with the virtual world than a true addictive process.[76] Gilbert et al., accordingly, required all their study participants to have had at least six months of Second Life (an online virtual world) virtual residency. Even with such a requirement, Gilbert et al.'s study still found that players with a longer length of Second Life virtual residence were less likely to report moderate or severe dependence than those with a shorter length of virtual residence.[77] On the other hand, however, according to Gilbert et al., it is not necessarily correct to conclude that an indulgent use of the Internet during the initial early period will definitely be successfully adjusted to a less indulgent or normal level of use later on. For example, Gentile reported that the average number of years playing video games for the pathological gamers in his study was 6.6 years ($SD = 3.2$) and it was 5.5 years ($SD = 3.2$) for the nonpathological gamers.[78]

The addicted individuals also spent significantly more time on sessions than their nonaddicted counterparts. For example, Zhou, Tang, and Peng found that the average time per week on line was 23.73 hours for the addicted group versus 7.57 hours for the nonaddicted group.[79] A study by Wang and colleagues in 2011 found that respondents who were using the Internet for more than eight hours a day were three times more likely to develop problematic Internet usage than their counterparts who were online for less than two hours a day.[80] Lin, Ko, and Wu's regression analysis showed that amount of time of Internet use per week independently associates with Internet addiction.[81]

Repeated exposures to or high amounts of Internet usage may precipitate Internet addiction, particularly among people who are genetically predisposed. Genetic environment interaction theory suggests that whether a genetic vulnerability is expressed mainly depends on whether it meets a vulnerable environment. Multiple factors may be involved regarding whether a susceptible person actually develops addiction, and one of the factors is repeated exposure to the substrate, which can be alcohol, gambling, or possibly the Internet.[82] However, one caveat is that many studies on this topic were not prospective but cross-sectional in nature and, therefore, the association between high amount of usage and Internet addiction could be bidirectional. In other words, the relationship could mean that a high amount of usage precipitates addiction or that addiction leads to a greater amount of usage, as Lin et al. state, ". . . it may be as much a symptom as it is a cause."[83]

Screening, Assessment, and Diagnosis

DSM-IV and *DSM-5* Diagnosis Categories

Internet use disorder is not a formal diagnosis in *DSM-IV*. Pies suggests that Internet addiction related symptoms can be placed under the section of Impulse Control Disorder Not Otherwise Specified (ICDNOS),[84] which is a subcategory of the category of Impulse Control Disorder Not Elsewhere Classified

(ICDNEC) in *DSM-IV*. He also suggests that clinicians might consider using "V" code of "phase of life problems" for their less severe cases of problematic Internet use, especially among young clients with issues related to developmental adjustment.[85]

Although the *DSM-5* working group initially seriously considered Internet addiction to meet the diagnostic inclusion criteria, the proposed draft of *DSM-5* released in 2012 (up to September) does not include it in a diagnostic category. Instead, Internet addiction or Internet use disorder was recommended by the work group to be placed in the *DSM-5* appendix to encourage more research.[86] While the *DSM-5* work groups did not include Internet Use Disorder as a formal diagnosis in the newly formed category of Substance Use and Addictive Disorders, they recommended nine criteria for further research in Section III.[87] The work groups did not state the number of criteria out of the nine that need to be met, but they indicated in their website that they will later recommend severity criteria. Furthermore, the nine criteria appear to be focused on Internet gaming. The nine criteria are (as of September 2012): a) preoccupied with Internet gaming; b) experiencing withdrawal symptoms without Internet; c) feeling the need to engage in a greater amount of Internet gaming; d) attempting to control the use of Internet gaming but without success; e) persisting extreme use of Internet despite awareness of negative psychosocial consequences; f) losing interest in previous hobbies and entertainment—with the exception of Internet gaming—because of excessive use of Internet gaming; g) using Internet gaming to alleviate dysphoric emotion; h) lying to significant others, therapist, or others about the extent of Internet gaming; and i) having jeopardized an important relationship, work, school or career opportunity as a result of Internet gaming use.

Internet Addiction or Pathological Internet Use Scales
Because Internet addiction is a relatively newer concept compared to substance addiction or other behavioral

addiction, such as pathological gambling, there is so far no "gold standard" with respect to its screening, assessment, and diagnosis. However, practitioners and researchers have been making efforts to establish valid and reliable scales to measure the risks and degree of Internet addiction, mostly by borrowing and modifying the criteria and other insights from the existing addiction literature, including the *DSM-IV* substance dependence criteria, the *DSM-IV* pathological gambling criteria, and others. By complying with the definition presented in *DSM-IV-TR* regarding the general impulse control disorders, Shapira and colleagues proposed the following widely cited three components, indicating essential diagnostic criteria for Internet addiction:

A. Maladaptive preoccupation with Internet use, as indicated by at least one of the following:

  1. Preoccupations with use of the Internet that are experienced as irresistible.

  2. Excessive use of the Internet for periods of time longer than planned.

B. The use of the Internet or the preoccupation with its use causes clinically significant distress or impairment in social, occupational, or other important areas of functioning.

C. The excessive Internet use does not occur exclusively during periods of hypomania or mania and is not better accounted for by other Axis I disorders.[88]

Currently, several scales are available to measure the risk of Internet addiction. Adapted from the *DSM-IV* pathological gambling diagnostic criteria, the Internet Addiction Test (IAT, see Appendix) has been one of the most used tools.[89] In answering the items on the IAT, clients should take into account only the time spent online for recreational or nonessential (i.e., nonacademic or nonjob) use purposes. The IAT contains twenty items, and each item has a five-point scale, ranging from one (rarely); two (occasionally); three (frequently); four (often); to five (always). A total score of twenty to forty-nine suggests an "average online user"; fifty to seventy-nine, a person is "experiencing occasional or frequent problems because of the Internet"; and eighty to 100 means the Internet usage of a person "is causing significant problems" in his or her life.

In addition to possessing validity and reliability, the advantages of IAT include that it can be filled out by the indexed persons or their significant others, that it helps identify which life area(s) the problematic Internet use has affected (e.g., sleep pattern, daily routine, productivity), and that its scoring system offers a continuum ranging from a minimum total score of twenty to a maximum total score of 100, as well as cutoff scores differentiating degree of severity. The quantitative nature of IAT is consistent with the *DSM-5*'s emphasis on assessing clients based on a continuum with cutoffs so that clinicians can evaluate whether a client is in the mild, moderate, severe, or very severe category, and can follow up on the client's progress.

Another quantitative-in-nature scale that also has validity and reliability is the Compulsive Internet Use Scale (CIUS) developed by Meerkerk and colleagues.[90] The items of CIUS are based on the *DSM-IV* substance dependence, *DSM-IV* pathological gambling, and Griffiths' insight on behavioral addiction. Compared with the IAT, the CIUS is a shorter instrument, with only fourteen items. Each item can be rated on a five-point scale, with zero being never; one (seldom); two (sometimes); three (often); and four (very often). The lowest total score a person can get is zero and the highest is fifty-six. The authors, however, did not suggest cut-off scores to differentiate severity. The term "Internet" in both the IAT and the CIUS can refer to all forms of online activity, such as Internet gaming, social network sites, chat room, online gambling, or cybersex. A copy of the CIUS is included in the Appendix.

Unlike the IAT and the CIUS, the Pathological Internet Use Scale (PIU), the Young's Diagnostic Questionnaire (YDQ), the Pathological Video-Game Use Scale (PVGUS), and the scale used by Grusser, Thalemann, and Griffiths to determine pathological gamers do not have a quantitative scoring system. Instead, they adopted a strategy more similar to the *DSM-IV*'s. In other words, the focus is whether a person should be rendered a diagnosis or not; degrees of severity of the symptoms or problems are not measured. A person would be given a diagnosis if he or she meets a certain number of the total criteria. For example, the *DSM-IV* defines a person as having pathological gambling disorder if he or she positively endorsed five of the ten criteria listed.

The PIU is a thirteen-item scale that measures evidence with respect to the negative effects of Internet use on various life areas such as personal distress, withdrawal symptoms, mood-altering use, interpersonal problems, academic, and work performance. The PIU determines a person a "pathological Internet user" if he or she ratifies four or more of the thirteen items.[91] The authors further categorized those who did not endorse any item as "No Symptoms," those with one to three items as "Limited Symptoms," and those with four or more, "pathological Internet user." The PIU has high internal reliability, but Morahan-Martin and Schumacher did not mention its validity.

According to Gentile, the eleven-item PVGUS is based on the *DSM-IV* Pathological Gambling criteria and shares basic characteristics with Brown's 1991 essential definition of addiction—the activity controls the individual's life; the activity provides pleasure or relieves unpleasant feelings; more of the activity is required to achieve the effect; the person experiences negative physical or mental effects when the activity is disengaged or stopped; the activity results in conflict with a job or other responsibilities or the relationships with other people; and the person continues engaging in the activity despite efforts to refrain from doing it. A gamer who shows at least six of the eleven symptoms will be considered as a pathological video game user. The PVGUS appears to have construct validity and reliability.[92]

Treatment

Treating Co-Occurring Disorders

As mentioned earlier, Internet addiction often co-occurs with other psychiatric disorders or impulse control disorder, such as depression, suicidal behavior, ADHD, anxiety, substance use disorders, or compulsive shopping. Regardless of whether such a co-occurrence involves a causal relationship, whether Internet addiction results in psychiatric symptoms, or whether Internet addiction functions as self-medication of the psychiatric symptoms, it is crucial to screen for, assess, and treat the occurring psychiatric disorders and symptoms when the primary presenting problem is Internet addiction, or vice versa. Shaw and Black suggest that when working with a client with Internet addiction, clinicians need to explore the client's past history of psychiatric disorders and treatment, including hospitalizations, medications, and psychotherapy.[93] A thorough coverage of all involved symptoms and disorders in treatment can enhance the treatment effectiveness of Internet addiction and prevent relapse.[94]

Adopting Total Abstinence and/or Moderated Use

Unlike quitting the use of alcohol and/or other drugs—in that total abstinence can be pursued without jeopardizing school or work—it is often practically unfeasible to ask an Internet addict to be totally abstinent from computer or Internet use in modern society, as school assignments and office work often require computer and Internet usage. To solve the dilemma, Young recommended that Internet addicts may adopt a) the total abstinence stance with respect only to a specific Internet application (e.g., a sex website, a chat room, an interactive video game), which actually triggers Internet binges and b) a moderated-use strategy with respect to the overall computer or Internet use.[95] Young's strategy would be feasible because the research has shown that most people are addicted to specific Internet applications, such as sex websites, interactive chat rooms, and gaming, not to the general Internet use for research or knowledge-searching purposes.[96, 97] Thus, it is necessary for practitioners to conduct a thorough screening and assessment during intake to identify the specific Internet application(s) that initiate Internet addiction. Total abstinence from the specific Internet application prevents triggers, and moderated use of the general Internet reduces the risk of relapse and still allows the individual to fulfill the stipulations of school and work.

Implementing Crisis Management: "First-Order" Changes

Citing Delmonico, Young states two levels of intervention and treatment of Internet sex addiction: the "first-order" changes focus on crisis management and the "second-order" changes target more long-term recovery.[98] These two levels of intervention and treatment not only can be applied to Internet sex addiction, but also to other types of Internet addictions.

The first-order changes may involve several concrete steps to reduce access to the computer or Internet use. A client can install filtering software and/or use some stimulants, such as an alarm clock or a sign near the computer, to prompt a limit to online time.[99] "Practicing the opposite" is another strategy; a client may replace his or her routine, nonstop Internet-using schedule (such as going online continuously from the moment arriving home from work to going to bed) with a new, less Internet-using addiction-prone schedule (such as chopping into the middle of the process by taking a break for dinner and watching TV and then returning to use).[100] "A reminder card" that lists, for example, five major drawbacks Internet addiction brought about and the five benefits from decreasing the use of the Internet can also be useful in promoting the client's controllable and responsible Internet use.[101]

Providing Cognitive Behavior Therapy: "Second-Order" Changes

Cognitive behavioral therapy (CBT) has been widely applied to help clients with substance use disorders or other impulse-control disorders such as pathological gambling, and CBT is also recommended to help clients with Internet addiction. CBT may help clients create "second-order" change necessary for long-term recovery.[102] CBT includes two major components: functional analysis and skills training. Functional analysis explores triggers (e.g., stress) that lead to a client's dysfunctional or maladaptive behavior (e.g., Internet bingeing), and the short-term beneficial consequences (e.g., escape) that reinforce the dysfunctional or maladaptive behavior. Skills training, on the other hand, helps the client develop useful coping skills or adaptive behaviors (e.g., jogging or applying other effective stress management skills, getting couple's therapy) to replace the old dysfunctional behavior (e.g., resorting to Internet binge) in responding to the triggers. It also reminds the client of the long-term negative consequences (e.g., time lost and the stressor remains) of adopting the dysfunctional behavior, so that the client's dysfunctional behavior will not be sustained through the reinforcement of the short-term benefit (e.g., a temporary escape of the stress).

Restructuring Distorted Thoughts. According to Young, cognitive restructuring is an important CBT component for helping Internet addicts.[103] Internet addicts tend to have distorted thoughts and believe that the virtual world treats them well, but the real world does not. They believe they can gain achievement and self-esteem from the virtual world, whereas in their real lives they do not have opportunities to achieve what they want to and their efforts are futile. Their all-or-nothing maladaptive cognition, such as "Nobody loves me offline . . . . The online game world is the only place where I am respected," or "I am worthless offline, but in the online world I am someone," often gives them permission to engage in Internet binges and intensify their Internet addiction.[104] Practitioners can help clients to be aware that a) reliance on the avatars and other involvements in the virtual world to fulfill the unmet needs in real lives is unhealthy because it only reinforces a temporary escape from issues encountered in real lives and will not actually solve the problems in life or produce authentic self-esteem; b) there are areas and opportunities in real life that people can invest in and pursue, with right strategies and efforts, to achieve their goals, increase their self-esteem, and satisfy their needs.

Transferring from Virtual to Reality. Although practitioners should encourage a client to leave or reduce exposure to the virtual world, paradoxically, entering a client's virtual world and examining the client's relationship to the avatar, as well as the virtual social links involved, helps a practitioner identify key issues the client may be experiencing and the needs he or she is longing to fulfill. This strategy is specifically relevant to helping younger addicted game players, who may often excessively engage in role-playing games to unknowingly compensate for some areas that are lacking in their real lives.[105] Practitioners learning what a virtual world provides to clients and its therapeutic function for them can provide insights and facilitate directions for both the practitioners and clients to work on to enrich clients' real lives and reduce their indulgence in the virtual world.[106]

Expanding Functional Coping Repertoire. Li, Wang, and Wang's 2009 study found that their problematic Internet use group tended to experience a higher level of stressful events during the past six months than their nonproblematic Internet use counterparts. Furthermore, the problematic Internet users also used more avoidant coping styles and less problem-solving styles than the nonproblematic Internet users.[107] Therefore, helping the client replace avoidant coping styles with functional copying skills can be beneficial. To expand the functional skills repertoire, practitioners can collaborate with clients and help them acquire time management skills and therefore better prioritize goals for which online time can be allocated efficiently and the amount of time online controlled; develop more functional coping skills based on their strengths and resources and tailored to fit their situations; expand their satisfying offline activities; and link them with supportive systems.[108] Young also encourages Internet addicts to fill out a personal inventory encompassing all the hobbies and activities they used to carry out but were now put aside or neglected because of their addiction to the Internet. This inventory can assist Internet addicts to reflect on the normal life activities they used to engage in and perhaps become motivated to resume those lost activities.[109]

Offering individual or group format of CBT. Nabuco de Abreu and Goes applied a group format of CBT—structured cognitive therapy—to help their Internet addicted clients.[110] The first step is to build therapeutic alliance between the group and the practitioners and relationships among group members. Group members are asked to keep a weekly diary logging their negative and unsatisfied emotional needs that lead them to pursue the virtual world in order to fulfill those needs. They specify the chain of their Internet addiction behavior, including the situations and events that trigger their craving for the Internet, the amount of time spent, and the accompanying thoughts and feelings. In each group session, one or two members share their situations; the group discusses these situations and the practitioner provides functional strategies for dealing with the situations when they occur again.

Involving Family-Oriented Treatment

A family may have contributed to or was a risk factor for an addict's addiction; to change the individual's addictive behavior, the entire family system may need to be reworked. Regardless of whether the family is the cause of an individual's addiction, family members tend to suffer from the addiction's negative consequences. Repairing the damaged relationship between the addict and the family and bringing the family back to serve as a supportive resource is critical for promoting the individual's recovery.

As mentioned previously in this chapter, numerous empirical studies have shown the connection between a dysfunctional family and an adolescent's indulging in Internet activities, such as online gaming. Empirical studies also show that family-based treatment improves family function and decreases adolescents' Internet addiction.[111, 112] For example, Zhong and colleagues found that a family-based treatment improves the Internet addiction among Chinese adolescents more effectively than a conventional treatment does. The family-based treatment included promoting family function and a supportive atmosphere, increasing accurate knowledge of Internet use, changing self-perception and facilitating self-confidence, and increasing hope for recovery. The conventional treatment adopted mainly military training, such as long-distance running, swimming, weightlifting, and group therapy targeting addictive behaviors.[113]

Various evidence-based family-oriented treatments are available to help substance-abusing adolescents—for example, the multidimensional family therapy (MDFT) and the brief strategic family therapy—and they may be applied to help Internet-addicted adolescents.[114, 115] The MDFT targets three domains: the adolescent, the parents (and other family members), and the interaction between the adolescent and the parents. Each session can begin with the adolescent alone and the parents alone followed by the joint family session. The MDFT individual sessions with the adolescent focus on facilitating engaging in treatment; enhancing cognitive understanding of the detrimental effects of the addictive behavior; strengthening coping skills, problem-solving ability, and functional alternative behavior in coping with triggers; and increasing association with prosocial peers.

Individual sessions with the parents focus on decreasing the parents' own substance-abusing behavior—in this case, examining their own Internet use behaviors and searching for ways to model appropriate Internet use. The sessions also focus on increasing the parents' resources and social support, and enhancing parenting practice—monitoring their child's Internet activities and other behavior, clarifying their expectations of the child, and setting rules with respect to Internet use.[116] The joint family sessions focus on parental commitment to the adolescent and the adolescent's attachment to the parents, with a goal of developing a positive parent-child relationship. A positive parent-child relationship is a prerequisite for effective parental monitoring of a child's Internet use; a child is less likely to comply with parental rules without a strong bond with the family and parents.

Family-oriented treatment is also crucial in the case of Internet sex or pornography addiction. Often, the spouse or significant other of an Internet sex addict experiences extreme shame, guilt, embarrassment, inadequacy, and even trauma after discovering the online sex addiction of their loved one.[117, 118] Family-oriented treatment or couple therapy, therefore, is necessary to start the healing process, which may directly or indirectly facilitate the recovery of the client and the family. To help a female partner of a man addicted to pornography, Bergner and Bridges suggest that a clinician should emphasize to the woman that the man's pornography addiction is not about her inadequacy but about his own struggle, such as his attempts to restore his damaged self-esteem or recover from sexual childhood degradations.

Degradation of the addicted partner needs to be minimized; instead of perceiving him as a "pervert," he should be viewed as a man in an irrational and pathological state. Partners should not attack the addicts or threaten the addicts or coerce them to change, as those behaviors have proved to be unsuccessful and will only worsen the existing problems.[119] Ford and colleagues further recommend structural family therapy (SFT) to help the couples. They said that pornography generates a new coalition with the addicted person and it weakens the couple's alliance and relationship. The goal of SFT is to create more opportunities for the couple to rebuild closeness and intimacy so that, rather than turning to outside sources to deal with problems, they can rely on each other, which will further reinforce a satisfying and intact relationship.[120]

Appendix

Internet Addiction Test (IAT)

How do you know if you're already addicted or rapidly tumbling toward trouble? The Internet Addiction Test is the first validated and reliable measure of addictive use of the Internet. Developed by Dr. Kimberly Young, the IAT is a 20-item questionnaire that measures mild, moderate, and severe levels of Internet Addiction.

To assess your level of addiction, answer the following questions using this scale:

1 = Rarely   2 = Occasionally   3 = Frequently   4 = Often   5 = Always

1. How often do you find that you stay on-line longer than you intended?

   ___ Rarely
   ___ Occasionally
   ___ Frequently
   ___ Often
   ___ Always
   ___ Does Not Apply

2. How often do you neglect household chores to spend more time on-line?

   ___ Rarely
   ___ Occasionally
   ___ Frequently
   ___ Often
   ___ Always
   ___ Does Not Apply

3. How often do you prefer the excitement of the Internet to intimacy with your partner?

   ___ Rarely
   ___ Occasionally
   ___ Frequently
   ___ Often
   ___ Always
   ___ Does Not Apply

4. How often do you form new relationships with fellow on-line users?

   ___ Rarely
   ___ Occasionally
   ___ Frequently
   ___ Often
   ___ Always
   ___ Does Not Apply

5. How often do others in your life complain to you about the amount of time you spend on-line?

   ___ Rarely
   ___ Occasionally
   ___ Frequently
   ___ Often
   ___ Always
   ___ Does Not Apply

6. How often do your grades or school work suffer because of the amount of time you spend on-line?

   ___ Rarely
   ___ Occasionally
   ___ Frequently
   ___ Often
   ___ Always
   ___ Does Not Apply

7. How often do you check your e-mail before something else that you need to do?

___ Rarely
___ Occasionally
___ Frequently
___ Often
___ Always
___ Does Not Apply

8. How often does your job performance or productivity suffer because of the Internet?

___ Rarely
___ Occasionally
___ Frequently
___ Often
___ Always
___ Does Not Apply

9. How often do you become defensive or secretive when anyone asks you what you do on-line?

___ Rarely
___ Occasionally
___ Frequently
___ Often
___ Always
___ Does Not Apply

10. How often do you block out disturbing thoughts about your life with soothing thoughts of the Internet?

___ Rarely
___ Occasionally
___ Frequently
___ Often
___ Always
___ Does Not Apply

11. How often do you find yourself anticipating when you will go on-line again?

___ Rarely
___ Occasionally
___ Frequently
___ Often
___ Always
___ Does Not Apply

12. How often do you fear that life without the Internet would be boring, empty, and joyless?

___ Rarely
___ Occasionally
___ Frequently
___ Often
___ Always
___ Does Not Apply

13. How often do you snap, yell, or act annoyed if someone bothers you while you are on-line?

___ Rarely
___ Occasionally
___ Frequently
___ Often
___ Always
___ Does Not Apply

14. How often do you lose sleep due to late-night log-ins?

___ Rarely
___ Occasionally
___ Frequently
___ Often
___ Always
___ Does Not Apply

15. How often do you feel preoccupied with the Internet when off-line, or fantasizing about being on-line?

___ Rarely
___ Occasionally
___ Frequently
___ Often
___ Always
___ Does Not Apply

16. How often do you find yourself saying "just a few more minutes" when on-line?

___ Rarely
___ Occasionally
___ Frequently
___ Often
___ Always
___ Does Not Apply

17. How often do you try to cut down the amount of time you spend on-line and fail?

___ Rarely
___ Occasionally
___ Frequently
___ Often
___ Always
___ Does Not Apply

18. How often do you try to hide how long you've been on-line?

___ Rarely
___ Occasionally
___ Frequently
___ Often
___ Always
___ Does Not Apply

19. How often do you choose to spend more time on-line over going out with others?

___ Rarely
___ Occasionally
___ Frequently
___ Often
___ Always
___ Does Not Apply

20. How often do you feel depressed, moody, or nervous when you are off-line, which goes away once you are back on-line?

___ Rarely
___ Occasionally
___ Frequently
___ Often
___ Always
___ Does Not Apply

Scoring:

Total the numbers for each response to obtain a final score. The higher your score, the greater your level of addiction and the problems your Internet usage causes. Here's a general scale to help measure your score:

20 – 49 points: You are an average on-line user. You may surf the Web a bit too long at times, but you have control over your usage.

50 – 79 points: You are experiencing occasional or frequent problems because of the Internet. You should consider their full impact on your life.

80 – 100 points: Your Internet usage is causing significant problems in your life. You should evaluate the impact of the Internet on your life and address the problems directly caused by your Internet usage.

After you have identified the category that fits your total score, look back at those questions for which you scored a 4 or 5. Did you realize this was a significant problem for you?

Dr. Kimberly S. Young, founder of the Center for Internet Addiction Recovery. This test is available at netaddiction.com. Used with permission.

Compulsive Internet Use Scale (CIUS)

The following questions should be answered about your use of the Internet for private purposes.

Answers can be given on a 5-point scale:

(0) Never, (1) Seldom, (2) Sometimes, (3) Often, (4) Very often.

1. How often do you find it difficult to stop using the Internet when you are online?

2. How often do you continue to use the Internet despite your intention to stop?

3. How often do others (e.g., partner, children, parents, friends) say you should use the Internet less?

4. How often do you prefer to use the Internet instead of spending time with others (e.g., partner, children, parents, friends)?

5. How often are you short of sleep because of the Internet?

6. How often do you think about the Internet, even when not online?

7. How often do you look forward to your next Internet session?

8. How often do you think you should use the Internet less often?

9. How often have you unsuccessfully tried to spend less time on the Internet?

10. How often do you rush through your (home) work in order to go on the Internet?

11. How often do you neglect your daily obligations (work, school, or family life) because you prefer to go on the Internet?

12. How often do you go on the Internet when you are feeling down?

13. How often do you use the Internet to escape from your sorrows or get relief from negative feelings?

14. How often do you feel restless, frustrated, or irritated when you cannot use the Internet?

Meerkerk, G. J., Van den Eijnden, R. J. J. M., Vermulst, A. A., and Garretsen, H. F. L. (2009). The Compulsive Internet Use Scale (CIUS): Some Psychometric Properties. Cyberpsychology & Behavior, 12(1), 1–6. Used with permission.

(HBI-19)

Date:_____
ID #: _____

Below are a number of statements that describe various thoughts, feelings, and behaviors. As you answer each question, circle the number on the right that best describes you. Only circle one number per statement and please be sure to answer every question.

For the purpose of this questionnaire, sex is defined as any activity or behavior that stimulates or arouses a person with the intent to produce an orgasm or sexual pleasure. _Sexual behaviors may or may not involve a partner_. (e.g. self-masturbation or solo-sex, using pornography, intercourse with a partner, oral sex, anal sex, etc…)

		Never	Rarely	Sometimes	Often	Very Often
1.	I use sex to forget about the worries of daily life.	1	2	3	4	5
2.	Even though I promised myself I would not repeat a sexual behavior, I find myself returning to it over and over again.	1	2	3	4	5
3.	Doing something sexual helps me feel less lonely.	1	2	3	4	5
4.	I engage in sexual activities that I know I will later regret.	1	2	3	4	5
5.	I sacrifice things I really want in life in order to be sexual.	1	2	3	4	5
6.	I turn to sexual activities when I experience unpleasant feelings (e.g. frustration, sadness, anger).	1	2	3	4	5
7.	My attempts to change my sexual behavior fail.	1	2	3	4	5
8.	When I feel restless, I turn to sex in order to soothe myself.	1	2	3	4	5
9.	My sexual thoughts and fantasies distract me from accomplishing important tasks.	1	2	3	4	5
10.	I do things sexually that are against my values and beliefs.	1	2	3	4	5
11.	Even though my sexual behavior is irresponsible or reckless I find it difficult to stop.	1	2	3	4	5
12.	I feel like my sexual behavior is taking me in a direction I don't want to go.	1	2	3	4	5
13.	Doing something sexual helps me cope with stress.	1	2	3	4	5
14.	My sexual behavior controls my life.	1	2	3	4	5
15.	My sexual cravings and desires feel stronger than my self-discipline.	1	2	3	4	5
16.	Sex provides a way for me to deal with emotional pain I feel.	1	2	3	4	5
17.	Sexually, I behave in ways I think are wrong.	1	2	3	4	5
18.	I use sex as a way to try and help myself deal with my problems.	1	2	3	4	5
19.	My sexual activities interfere with aspects of my life such as work or school.	1	2	3	4	5

Rory C. Reid, Ph.D., Department of Psychiatry and Biobehavioral Sciences, University of California, Los Angeles
Sheila Garos, Ph.D., Psychology Department, Texas Tech University
Bruce N. Carpenter, Ph.D., Department of Psychology, Brigham Young University

COPE: 1.3.6.8.13.16.18   CONSO: 5.9.14.19   CTRL: 2.4.7.10.11.12.15.17

Eating Attitudes Test (EAT-26)

Age: _____   Current Weight: _____   Highest weight (excluding
pregnancy): _____
Sex: _____
Height: _____   Lowest Adult Weight: _____   Ideal Weight: _____

✓ Please choose one response by marking a check to the right for each of the following statements:	Always	Usually	Often	Some times	Rarely	Never	Score
1. Am terrified about being overweight.							
2. Avoid eating when I am hungry.							
3. Find myself preoccupied with food.							
4. Have gone on eating binges where I feel that I may not be able to stop.							
5. Cut my food into small pieces.							
6. Aware of the calorie content of foods that I eat.							
7. Particularly avoid food with a high carbohydrate content (i.e. bread, rice, potatoes, etc.)							
8. Feel that others would prefer if I ate more.							
9. Vomit after I have eaten.							
10. Feel extremely guilty after eating.							
11. Am preoccupied with a desire to be thinner.							
12. Think about burning up calories when I exercise.							
13. Other people think that I am too thin.							
14. Am preoccupied with the thought of having fat on my body.							
15. Take longer than others to eat my meals.							
16. Avoid foods with sugar in them.							
17. Eat diet foods.							
18. Feel that food controls my life.							
19. Display self-control around food.							
20. Feel that others pressure me to eat.							
21. Give too much time and thought to food.							
22. Feel uncomfortable after eating sweets.							
23. Engage in dieting behavior.							
24. Like my stomach to be empty.							
25. Have the impulse to vomit after meals.							
26. Enjoy trying new rich foods.							
Total Score =							

Behavioral Questions:

In the past 6 months have you:	Yes	No
A. Gone on eating binges where you feel that you may not be able to stop? (Eating much more than most people would eat under the same circumstances) If you answered yes, how often during the worst week: _____		
B. Ever made yourself sick (vomited) to control your weight or shape? If you answered yes, how often during the worst week: _____		
C. Ever used laxatives, diet pills or diuretics (water pills) to control your weight or shape? If you answered yes, how often during the worst week? _____		
D. Ever been treated for an eating disorder? When: _____		

EAT-26 From: Garner et al. 1982, *Psychological Medicine, 12,* 871-878); adapted by D. Garner with permission.

Note: For more information on the EAT-26, see: www.river-centre.org

SCORING THE EATING ATTITUDES TEST (EAT-26) ©

Follow the 5 steps below:

Step 1: EAT-26 ITEM SCORING:	
Score each item as indicated below and put score in box to the right of each item	

Items # 1-25:			Item #26 only:	
Always	=	3	=	0
Usually	=	2	=	0
Often	=	1	=	0
Sometimes	=	0	=	1
Rarely	=	0	=	2
Never	=	0	=	3

Step 2: Total EAT-26 Score	
	Total =
Add item scores together for a Total EAT-26 score:	

Step 3: Behavioral Questions	
	Yes
Did you score Yes on Questions A, B, C or D?	

Step 4: Underweight
Determine if you are significantly underweight according to the table to the right

Step 5: Referral	No	Yes
If your EAT-26 score is **20 or more**		
or if you answered **YES** to any questions A-D		
or if your **weight** is below the number on the weight chart to the right,		
Please discuss your results with your physician or therapist		

Significantly Underweight According to Height
(Body Mass Index of 18)*

Height (inches)	Weight (pounds)	Height (inches)	Weight (pounds)
58	86	68	118
58	88	68	120
59	89	69	121
59	90	69	124
60	91	70	125
60	93	70	127
61	95	71	128
61	96	71	131
62	99	72	132
62	100	72	134
63	101	73	135
63	103	73	138
64	105	74	140
64	106	74	141
65	108	75	144
65	109	75	146
66	112	76	147
66	113	76	149
67	114	77	152
67	117	77	154

* Note: The table above indicates the body weights for heights considered to be "significantly underweight" according to a Body Mass Index (BMI) of 18. BMI is a simple method of evaluating body weight taking height into consideration. It applies to both men and women. There is some controversy regarding whether or not BMI is the best method of determining relative body weight and it is important to recognize that it is possible for someone to be quite malnourished even though they are above the weight listed in the table. In order to determine if you are "significantly underweight", locate your height (without shoes) on the table and see if the corresponding body weight (in light indoor clothing) is below that listed. If so, you are considered "significantly underweight" and should speak to your physician or therapist about your weight. To Calculate Body Mass Index (BMI) exactly: Weight (pounds) Divided by Height in Inches; Divide this again by Height in Inches and Multiply by 703
BMI = (lbs) ÷ (inches) ÷ (inches) X 703

Eating Attitudes Test (EAT-26)

The following screening questionnaire is designed to help you determine if your eating behaviors and attitudes warrant further evaluation. The questionnaire is **not intended to provide a diagnosis**. Rather, it identifies the presence of symptoms that are consistent with either a possible eating disorder.

Answer the questions as honestly as you can, and then score questions using the instructions at the end.

✓ Please mark a check to the right of each of the following statements:	Always	Usually	Often	Some times	Rarely	Never	Score
1. Am terrified about being overweight.							
2. Avoid eating when I am hungry.							
3. Find myself preoccupied with food.							
4. Have gone on eating binges where I feel that I may not be able to stop.							
5. Cut my food into small pieces.							
6. Aware of the calorie content of foods that I eat.							
7. Particularly avoid food with a high carbohydrate content (i.e. bread, rice, potatoes, etc.)							
8. Feel that others would prefer if I ate more.							
9. Vomit after I have eaten.							
10. Feel extremely guilty after eating.							
11. Am preoccupied with a desire to be thinner.							
12. Think about burning up calories when I exercise.							
13. Other people think that I am too thin.							
14. Am preoccupied with the thought of having fat on my body.							
15. Take longer than others to eat my meals.							
16. Avoid foods with sugar in them.							
17. Eat diet foods.							
18. Feel that food controls my life.							
19. Display self-control around food.							
20. Feel that others pressure me to eat.							
21. Give too much time and thought to food.							
22. Feel uncomfortable after eating sweets.							
23. Engage in dieting behavior.							
24. Like my stomach to be empty.							
25. Have the impulse to vomit after meals.							
26. Enjoy trying new rich foods.							
						Total Score=	

1) Have you gone on eating binges where you feel that you may not be able to stop?
(Eating much more than most people would eat under the same circumstances)
    _ No _ Yes How many times in the last 6 months? _____

2) Have you ever made yourself sick (vomited) to control your weight or shape?
    _ No _ Yes How many times in the last 6 months? _____

3) Have you ever used laxatives, diet pills or diuretics (water pills) to control your weight or shape?
    _ No _ Yes How many times in the last 6 months? _____

4) Have you ever been treated for an eating disorder? _ No _ Yes **When?** _____

EAT-26 ' David M. Garner (1982) Note: The EAT-26 has been made available with permission of the authors.

SCORING THE EATING ATTITUDES TEST (EAT-26)

Follow the steps below:

Step 1

EAT-26 ITEM SCORING:

Score each item as indicated below and put score in box to the right of each item

Items # 1-25:		Item #26 only:	
Always	= 3	=	0
Usually	= 2	=	0
Often	= 1	=	0
Sometimes	= 0	=	1
Rarely	= 0	=	2
Never	= 0	=	3

Step 2

Add item scores together for a Total EAT-26 score:	Total =

Step 3

Determine if you are significantly underweight according to the table to the right

Step 4

If your EAT-26 score is 20 or more or if your weight is below the number on the weight chart to the right, we suggest that you discuss your results with your physician or therapist

Significantly Underweight According to Height
(Body Mass Index of 18)*

Height (inches)	Weight (pounds)	Height (inches)	Weight (pounds)
58	86	68	118
58 _	88	68 _	120
59	89	69	121
59 _	90	69 _	124
60	91	70	125
60 _	93	70 _	127
61	95	71	128
61 _	96	71 _	131
62	99	72	132
62 _	100	72 _	134
63	101	73	135
63 _	103	73 _	138
64	105	74	140
64 _	106	74 _	141
65	108	75	144
65 _	109	75 _	146
66	112	76	147
66 _	113	76 _	149
67	114	77	152
67 _	117	77 _	154

* Note: The table above indicates the body weights for heights considered to be significantly underweight according to a Body Mass Index (BMI) of 18. BMI is a simple method of evaluating body weight taking height into consideration. It applies to both men and women. There is some controversy regarding whether or not BMI is the best method of determining relative body weight and it is important to recognize that it is possible for someone to be quite malnourished even though they are above the weight listed in the table. In order to determine if you are significantly underweight , locate your height (without shoes) on the table and see if the corresponding body weight (in light indoor clothing) is below that listed. If so, you are considered significantly underweight and should speak to your physician or therapist about your weight. To Calculate Body Mass Index (BMI) exactly: Weight (pounds) Divided by Height in Inches; Divide this again by Height in Inches and Multiply by 703
BMI = (lbs) (inches) (inches) X 703

The EAT-26 has been reproduced with permission. Garner et al. (1982).
The Eating Attitudes Test: Psychometric features and clinical correlates.
Psychological Medicine, 12, 871-878.

SEXUAL ADDICTION
SCREENING TEST – Revised
(SAST-R)

Name _____

Patient ID No. _____

Age _____ Male/Female _____ State _____

Therapist or Physician _____

SAST- R 2.0

The Sexual Addiction Screening Test (SAST) is designed to assist in the assessment of sexually compulsive or "addictive" behavior. Developed in cooperation with hospitals, treatment programs, private therapists and community groups, the SAST provides a profile of responses which help to discriminate between addictive and non-addictive behavior. To complete the test, answer each question by placing a check in the appropriate yes/no column.

❑ YES ❑ NO   1. Were you sexually abused as a child or adolescent?

❑ YES ❑ NO   2. Did your parents have trouble with sexual behavior?

❑ YES ❑ NO   3. Do you often find yourself preoccupied with sexual thoughts?

❑ YES ❑ NO   4. Do you feel that your sexual behavior is not normal?

❑ YES ❑ NO   5. Do you ever feel bad about your sexual behavior?

❑ YES ❑ NO   6. Has your sexual behavior ever created problems for you and your family?

❑ YES ❑ NO   7. Have you ever sought help for sexual behavior you did not like?

❑ YES ❑ NO   8. Has anyone been hurt emotionally because of your sexual behavior?

❑ YES ❑ NO   9. Are any of your sexual activities against the law?

❑ YES ❑ NO   10. Have you made efforts to quit a type of sexual activity and failed?

❑ YES ❑ NO   11. Do you hide some of your sexual behaviors from others?

❑ YES ❑ NO   12. Have you attempted to stop some parts of your sexual activity?

❑ YES ❑ NO   13. Have you felt degraded by your sexual behaviors?

❑ YES ❑ NO   14. When you have sex, do you feel depressed afterwards?

❑ YES ❑ NO   15. Do you feel controlled by your sexual desire?

❑ YES ❑ NO   16. Have important parts of your life (such as job, family, friends, leisure activities) been neglected because you were spending too much time on sex?

❑ YES ❑ NO   17. Do you ever think your sexual desire is stronger than you are?

❑ YES ❑ NO   18. Is sex almost all you think about?

❑ YES ❑ NO   19. Has sex (or romantic fantasies) been a way for you to escape your problems?

❑ YES ❑ NO   20. Has sex become the most important thing in your life?

❑ YES ❑ NO   21. Are you in crisis over sexual matters?

❑ YES ❑ NO   22. The internet has created sexual problems for you.

❑ YES ❑ NO   23. I spend too much time online for sexual purposes.

❑ YES ❑ NO 24. I have purchased services online for erotic purposes (sites for dating, pornography, fantasy and friend finder).

❑ YES ❑ NO 25. I have used the internet to make romantic or erotic connections with people online.

❑ YES ❑ NO 26. People in my life have been upset about my sexual activities online.

❑ YES ❑ NO 27. I have attempted to stop my online sexual behaviors.

❑ YES ❑ NO 28. I have subscribed to or regularly purchased or rented sexually explicit materials (magazines, videos, books or online pornography).

❑ YES ❑ NO 29. I have been sexual with minors.

❑ YES ❑ NO 30. I have spent considerable time and money on strip clubs, adult bookstores and movie houses.

❑ YES ❑ NO 31. I have engaged prostitutes and escorts to satisfy my sexual needs.

❑ YES ❑ NO 32. I have spent considerable time surfing pornography online.

❑ YES ❑ NO 33. I have used magazines, videos or online pornography even when there was considerable risk of being caught by family members who would be upset by my behavior.

❑ YES ❑ NO 34. I have regularly purchased romantic novels or sexually explicit magazines.

❑ YES ❑ NO 35. I have stayed in romantic relationships after they became emotionally abusive.

❑ YES ❑ NO 36. I have traded sex for money or gifts.

❑ YES ❑ NO 37. I have maintained multiple romantic or sexual relationships at the same time.

❑ YES ❑ NO 38. After sexually acting out, I sometimes refrain from all sex for a significant period.

❑ YES ❑ NO 39. I have regularly engaged in sadomasochistic behavior.

❑ YES ❑ NO 40. I visit sexual bath-houses, sex clubs or video/bookstores as part of my regular sexual activity.

❑ YES ❑ NO 41. I have engaged in unsafe or "risky" sex even though I knew it would cause me harm.

❑ YES ❑ NO 42. I have cruised public restrooms, rest areas or parks looking for sex with strangers.

❑ YES ❑ NO 43. I believe casual or anonymous sex has kept me from having more long-term intimate relationships.

❑ YES ❑ NO 44. My sexual behavior has put me at risk for arrest for lewd conduct or public indecency.

❑ YES ❑ NO 45. I have been paid for sex.

Core Item Scale	Questions 1-20	(Over 6)	_____

Subscales:

Internet Items	Questions 22-27	(3 or more)	_____
Men's Items	Questions 28-33	(2 or more)	_____
Women's Items	Questions 34-39	(2 or more)	_____
Homosexual Men	Questions 40-45	(3 or more)	_____

Addictive Dimensions:

Preoccupation   (2 or more)   _____
Items 3, 18, 19 and 20

Loss of Control   (2 or more)   _____
Items 10, 12, 15 and 17

Relationship Disturbance   (2 or more)   _____
Items 6, 8, 16 and 26

Affect Disturbance   (2 or more)   _____
Items 4, 5, 11, 13 and 14

Associated Features (not rated as a subscale)
Items 1, 2, 7, 9 and 21

Relative Distributions of
Addict & Nonaddict SAST Scores

This instrument has been based on screenings of tens of thousands of people. This particular version is a developmental stage revision of the instrument, so scoring may be adjusted with more research. Please be aware that clinical decisions must be made conditionally since final scoring protocols may vary.

BEHAVIORAL ADDICTION

SOUTH OAKS GAMBLING SCREEN (SOGS)

1. Indicate which of the following types of gambling you have done in your lifetime. For each type, mark one answer: "not at all," "less than once a week," or "once a week or more."

Not at all	Less than once a week	Once a week or more	
			a. played cards for money
			b. bet on horses, dogs or other animals (in off-track betting, at the track or with a bookie)
			c. bet on sports (parley cards, with a bookie, or at jai alai)
			d. played dice games (including craps, over and under, or other dice games) for money
			e. went to casino (legal or otherwise)
			f. played the numbers or bet on lotteries
			g. played bingo
			h. played the stock and/or commodities market
			i. played slot machines, poker machines or other gambling machines
			j. bowled, shot pool, played golf or played some other game of skill for money

2. What is the largest amount of money you have ever gambled with any one day?

____ never have gambled

____ more than $100 up to $1000

____ $10 or less

____ more than $1000 up to $10,000

____ more than $10 up to $100

____ more than $10,000

3. Do (did) your parents have a gambling problem?

____ both my father and mother gamble (or gambled) too much

____ my father gambles (or gambled) too much

____ my mother gambles (or gambled) too much

____ neither gambles (or gambled) too much

1

4. When you gamble, how often do you go back another day to win back money you lost?

____ never

____ some of the time (less than half the time) I lost

____ most of the time I lost

____ every time I lost

5. Have you ever claimed to be winning money gambling but weren't really? In fact, you lost?

____ never (or never gamble)

____ yes, less than half the time I lost

____ yes, most of the time

6. Do you feel you have ever had a problem with gambling?

____ no

____ yes, in the past, but not now

____ yes

	Yes	No
7. Did you ever gamble more than you intended?		
8. Have people criticized your gambling?		
9. Have you ever felt guilty about the way you gamble or what happens when you gamble?		
10. Have you ever felt like you would like to stop gambling but didn't think you could?		
11. Have you ever hidden betting slips, lottery tickets, gambling money, or other signs of gambling from your spouse, children, or other important people in you life?		
12. Have you ever argued with people you like over how you handle money?		
13. (If you answered "yes" to question 12): **Have money arguments ever centered on your gambling?**		
14. Have you ever borrowed from someone and not paid them back as a result of your gambling?		

	Yes	No
15. Have you ever lost time from work (or school) due to gambling?	――	――
16. If you borrowed money to gamble or to pay gambling debts, where did you borrow from? (Check "yes" or "no" for each)	――	――

	Yes	No
a. from household money		
b. from your spouse		
c. from other relatives or in-laws		
d. from banks, loan companies or credit unions		
e. from credit cards		
f. from loan sharks (Shylocks)		
g. your cashed in stocks, bonds or other securities		
h. you sold personal or family property		
i. you borrowed on your checking account (passed bad checks)		
j. you have (had) a credit line with a bookie		
k. you have (had) a credit line with a casino		

Scoring Rules for SOGS

Scores are determined by adding up the number of questions that show an "at risk" response, indicated as follows. If you answer the questions above with one of the following answers, mark that in the space next to that question:

Questions 1-3 are not counted

____ Question 4: most of the time I lost, or every time I lost

____ Question 5: yes, less than half the time I lose, or yes, most of the time

____ Question 6: yes, in the past, but not now, or yes

____ Question 7: yes

____ Question 8: yes

____ Question 9: yes

____ Question 10: yes

____ Question 11: yes

Question 12 is not counted

____ Question 13: yes

____ Question 14: yes

____ Question 15: yes

____ Question 16a: yes

____ Question 16b: yes

____ Question 16c: yes

____ Question 16d: yes

____ Question 16e: yes

____ Question 16f: yes

____ Question 16g: yes

____ Question 16h: yes

____ Question 16i: yes

Questions 16j and 16k are not counted

Total = _____ (20 questions are counted)

**3 or 4 = Potential pathological gambler (Problem gambler)

**5 or more = Probable pathological gambler

SOUTH OAKS GAMBLING SCREEN: REVISED FOR ADOLESCENTS (SOGS-RA)

The 12 scored items for the SOGS-RA from Winters, K.C., Stinchfield R.D. and Fulkerson, J. (1993a) are listed below.

a. How often have you gone back another day to try and win back money you lost gambling?

Every time/Most of the time/Some of the time/Never

b. When you were betting, have you ever told others you were winning money when you weren't?

Yes/No

c. Has your betting money ever caused any problems for you such as arguments with family and friends, or problems at school or work?

Yes/No

d. Have you ever gambled more than you had planned to?

Yes/No

e. Has anyone criticized your betting, or told you that you had a gambling problem whether you thought it true or not?

Yes/No

f. Have you ever felt bad about the amount of money you bet, or about what happens when you bet money?

Yes/No

g. Have you ever felt like you would like to stop betting, but didn't think you could?

Yes/No

h. Have you ever hidden from family or friends any betting slips, IOUs, lottery tickets, money that you won, or any signs of gambling?

Yes/No

i. Have you had money arguments with family or friends that centered on gambling?

Yes/No

j. Have you borrowed money to bet and not paid it back?

Yes/No

k. Have you ever skipped or been absent from school or work due to betting activities?

Yes/No

l. Have you borrowed money or stolen something in order to bet or to cover gambling activities?

Yes/No

Scoring Rules for SOGS-RA

Each item is scored either 1 (affirmative) or 0 (nonaffirmative). Item "a" is scored 1 if respondent indicates "every time" or "most of the time" and is scored 0 otherwise. Calculations for broad and narrow rates come from Winters, Stinchfield and Kim, 1995.

Calculation of Narrow Rates	Calculation of Broad Rates
Level 0 = No past year gambling.	Level 0 = No past year gambling
Level 1 = SOGS-RA score of _ 1	Level 1 = Gambling less than daily and SOGS-RA score = 0, OR, less than weekly gambling and SOGS-RA score _ 1.
Level 2 = SOGS-RA score of 2 or 3	Level 2 = At least weekly gambling and SOGS-RA score _ 1 OR gambling less than weekly and SOGS-RA score _ 2.
Level 3 = SOGS-RA score of _ 4	Level 3= At least weekly gambling + SOGS-RA score _ 2 OR daily gambling

Winters, K.C., Stinchfield, R.D, & Fulkerson, J. (1993). Toward the development of an adolescent problem severity scale. Journal of Gambling Studies, 9, 63-84.

Chapter Notes

CHAPTER ONE

1 Jeffrey L. Fortuna, "The obesity epidemic and food addiction: Clinical similarities to drug dependence," *Journal of Psychoactive Drugs* 44, no. 1 (2012): 56–63.

2 Ibid.

3 Nora D. Volkow and Roy A. Wise, "How can drug addiction help us understand obesity?" *Nature Neuroscience* 8 (2005): 555–60.

4 Nora D. Volkow, Bruce Rosen, and Lars Farde, "Imaging the living human brain: Magnetic resonance imaging and positron emission tomography," *Proceedings of the National Academy of Sciences of the United States of America* 94 (1997): 2787–88.

5 American Psychiatric Association, *Diagnostic and Statistical Manual of Mental Disorders, Fourth Edition, Text Revision* (Washington, DC: American Psychiatric Association, 2000).

6 Allen J. Frances and Thomas Widiger, "Psychiatric diagnosis: Lessons from the DSM–IV past and cautions for the DSM–5 future," *Annual Review of Clinical Psychology* 8 (2012): 109–30.

Ronald Pies, "Should DSM–V designate "Internet addiction" a mental disorder?" *Psychiatry* 6, no. 2 (2009): 31–37.

Nancy, M. Petry, "Commentary on Van Rooij et al. (2011): 'Gaming addiction'—a psychiatric disorder or not?" *Addiction* 106, no. 1 (2011): 213.

Howard Markel, "The D.S.M. gets addiction right," *The New York Times*, June 5, 2012, http://www.nytimes.com/2012/06/06/opinion/the-dsm-gets-addiction-right.html (accessed September 19, 2012).

7 American Society of Addiction Medicine, "The definition of addiction (adoption date: April 12, 2011)," http://www.asam.org/advocacy/find-a-policy-statement/view-policy-statement/public-policy-statements/2011/12/15/the-definition-of-addiction (accessed September 23, 2012).

8 Ibid.

9 National Institute on Drug Abuse, "Drugs, brains and behaviors: The science of addiction" (2010), http://www.drugabuse.gov/publications/media-guide/science-drug-abuse-addiction (accessed October 19, 2012).

10 Steve Sussman and Alan N. Sussman, "Considering the definition of addiction," *International Journal of Environmental Research and Public Health* 8 (2011): 4025.

11 American Psychiatric Association, *Diagnostic and Statistical Manual of Mental Disorders, Fourth Edition, Text Revision* (Washington, DC: American Psychiatric Association, 2000).

12 Ibid.

13 Ibid.

14 Ibid.

15 Jon E. Grant, Marc N. Potenza, Aviv Weinstein, and David A. Gorelick, "Introduction to Behavioral Addictions," *American Journal of Drug Alcohol Abuse* 36, no. 5 (2010): 233–41.

16 Christine Lochner, Dan J. Stein, Douglas Woods, David L. Pauls, Martin E. Franklin, Elizabeth H. Loerke, and Nancy J. Keuthen, "The validity of DSM-IV-TR criteria B and C or hair-pulling disorder (trichotillomania): Evidence from a clinical study," *Psychiatry Research* 189, no. 2 (2011): 276–80.

17 Leonardo F. Fontenelle, Sanne Oostermeijer, Ben J. Harrison, Christos Pantelis, and Murat Yucel, "Obsessive-compulsive disorder, impulse control disorders and drug addiction," *Drugs* 71, no. 7 (2011): 827–40.

18 Marc N. Potenza, Lorrin M. Koran, and Stefano Pallanti, "The relationship between impulse-control disorders and obsessive-compulsive disorder: A current understanding and future research directions," *Psychiatry Research* 170, no. 1 (2009): 22–31.

19 American Psychiatric Association, *Diagnostic and Statistical Manual of Mental Disorders, Fourth Edition, Text Revision* (Washington, DC: American Psychiatric Association, 2000).

20 Jon E. Grant, Marc N. Potenza, Aviv Weinstein, and David A. Gorelick, "Introduction to behavioral addictions," *American Journal of Drug and Alcohol Abuse* 36, no. 5 (2010): 233–41.

21 American Psychiatric Association, *Diagnostic and Statistical Manual of Mental Disorders, Fourth Edition, Text Revision* (Washington, DC: American Psychiatric Association, 2000).

22 R. Andrew Chambers, Jane R. Taylor, Marc N. Potenza, "Developmental neurocircuitry of motivation in adolescence: A critical period of addiction vulnerability," *American Journal of Psychiatry* 160, no. 6, (2003): 1041–52.

23 Jon E. Grant, *Impulse Control Disorders: A Clinician's Guide to Understanding and Treating Behavioral Addictions* (New York: W. W. Norton & Company, 2008).

24 Ibid.

25 Leonardo F. Fontenelle, Sanne Oostermeijer, Ben J. Harrison, Christos Pantelis, and Murat Yucel, "Obsessive-compulsive disorder, impulse control disorders and drug addiction," *Drugs* 71, no. 7 (2011): 827–40.

26 Ibid.

27 Himani Kashyap, Leonardo F. Fontenelle, Euripedes C. Miguel, Ygor A.

Ferrao, Albina R. Torres, Roseli G. Shavitt, Rafael Ferreira-Garcia, Maria C. do Rosario, and Murat Yucel, "Impulsive compulsivity in obsessive-compulsive disorder: A phenotypic marker of patients with poor clinical outcome," *Journal of Psychiatric Research* 46 (2012): 1146–52.

28 Jon E. Grant, *Impulse Control Disorders: A Clinician's Guide to Understanding and Treating Behavioral Addictions.* New York: W. W. Norton & Company, 2008.

29 American Psychiatric Association, "*DSM–5 Development.*" http://www.dsm5.org/proposedrevision/Pages/SubstanceUseandAddictiveDisorders.aspx (accessed September 19, 2012).

30 Ibid.

31 American Psychiatric Association, "*DSM–5 Development.*" http://www.dsm5.org/proposedrevision/Pages/SexualDysfunctions.aspx (accessed September 19, 2012).

32 Donald W. Black, Martha Shaw, and Nancee Blum, "Pathological gambling and compulsive buying: Do they fall within an obsessive-compulsive spectrum?" *Dialogues in Clinical Neuroscience* 12, no. 2 (2010): 175–85.

33 American Psychiatric Association, "*DSM–5 Development.*" http://www.dsm5.org/proposedrevision/Pages/SubstanceUseandAddictiveDisorders.aspx (accessed September 19, 2012).

34 Allen Frances, "DSM5 in Distress: DSM5 "Addiction" swallows substance abuse," *Psychology Today*, March 25, 2010, http://www.psychologytoday.com/blog/dsm5-in-distress/201003/dsm5-addiction-swallows-substance-abuse (accessed September 22, 2012).

35 American Psychiatric Association, "*DSM–5 Development.*" http://www.dsm5.org/ProposedRevision/Pages/proposedrevision.aspx?rid=452 (accessed September 22, 2012).

36 American Psychiatric Association, "*DSM–5 Development,*" http://www.dsm5.org/ProposedRevision/Pages/proposedrevision.aspx?rid=210 (accessed September 22, 2012).

37 George B. Mitzner, James P. Whelan, and Andrew W. Meyers, "Comments from the Trenches: Proposed changes to the DSM-V classification of pathological gambling," *Journal of Gambling Studies* 27 (2011): 517–21.

38 Daria J. Kuss and Mark D. Griffiths, "Internet and gaming addiction: A systematic literature review of neuroimaging studies," *Brain Sciences* 2, no. 3 (2012): 347–74.

39 Howard J. Shaffer, "Shifting perspectives on gambling and addiction," *Journal of Gambling Studies* 19, no. 1 (2003): 1–6.

40 Constance Holden, "'Behavioral' Addictions: Do they exist?" *Science* 294, no. 5544 (2001): 980–82.

41 David C. Hodgins, Jonathan N. Stea, and Jon E. Grant, "Gambling disorders," *Lancet* 378 (2011): 1874–84.

42 Jon E. Grant, *Impulse Control Disorders: A Clinician's Guide to Understanding and Treating Behavioral Addictions* (New York: W. W. Norton & Company, 2008).

43 Ibid.

44 David C. Hodgins, Jonathan N. Stea, and Jon E. Grant, "Gambling disorders," *Lancet* 378 (2011): 1874–84.

45 Jon E. Grant, Brian L. Odlaug, and Suck Won Kim, "Kleptomania: Clinical characteristics and relationship to substance use disorders," *The American Journal of Drug and Alcohol Abuse* 36, no. 5 (2010): 291–95.

46 Donald W. Black, Patrick O. Monahan, M'Hamed Temkit, and Martha Shaw,

"A family study of pathological gambling," *Psychiatry Research* 141 (2006): 295–303.

47 Jon E. Grant, *Impulse Control Disorders: A Clinician's Guide to Understanding and Treating Behavioral Addictions* (New York: W. W. Norton & Company, 2008).

48 Jon E. Grant, Marc N. Potenza, Aviv Weinstein, and David A. Gorelick, "Introduction to behavioral addictions," *American Journal of Drug and Alcohol Abuse* 36, no. 5 (2010): 233–41.

49 Jon E. Grant and Suck Won Kim, "Medication management of pathological gambling," *Minnesota Medicine* 89, no. 9 (2006): 44–48.

Nancy C. Raymond and Jon E. Grant, "Augmentation with naltrexone to treat compulsive sexual behavior: A case series," *Annals of Clinical Psychiatry* 22, no. 1 (2010): 56–62.

Ralph S. Ryback, "Naltrexone in the treatment of adolescent sexual offenders," *Journal of Clinical Psychiatry* 65, no. 7 (2004): 982–86.

Jon E. Grant, Suck Won Kim, and Brian L. Odlaug, "A double-blind, placebo-controlled study of the opiate antagonist, naltrexone, in the treatment of kleptomania," *Biological Psychiatry* 65, no. 7 (2009): 600–06.

50 American Psychiatric Association, "*DSM–5 Development.*" http://www.dsm5.org/proposedrevision/Pages/Obsessive-CompulsiveandRelatedDisorders.aspx (accessed September 21, 2012).

51 American Psychiatric Association, "*DSM–5 Development,*" http://www.dsm5.org/ProposedRevision/Pages/proposedrevision.aspx?rid=211# (accessed September 21, 2012).

52 Randy O. Frost and Tamara L. Hartl, "A cognitive-behavioral model of compulsive hoarding," *Behaviour Research and Therapy* 34 (1996): 341–50.

53 American Psychiatric Association, "*DSM–5 Development.*" http://www.dsm5.org/ProposedRevision/Pages/proposedrevision.aspx?rid=398# (accessed September 21, 2012).

54 American Psychiatric Association, "*DSM–5 Development.*" http://www.dsm5.org/ProposedRevision/Pages/proposedrevision.aspx?rid=211# (accessed September 21, 2012).

55 American Psychiatric Association, "*DSM–5 Development.*" http://www.dsm5.org/ProposedRevision/Pages/proposedrevision.aspx?rid=401# (accessed September 21, 2012.

56 Bernardo Dell'Osso, A. Carlo Altamura, Andrea Allen, Donatella Marazziti, and Eric Hollander, "Epidemiologic and clinical updates on impulse control disorders: A critical review," *European Archives of Psychiatry and Clinical Neuroscience* 256 (2006): 464–75.

57 Eric Hollander, Suah Kim, Ashley Braun, Daphne Simeon, and Joseph Zohar, "Cross-cutting issues and future directions for the OCD spectrum," *Psychiatry Research* 170 (2009): 3–6.

58 Marc N. Potenza, Lorrin M. Koran, and Stefano Pallanti, "The relationship between impulse-control disorders and obsessive-compulsive disorder: A current understanding and future research directions," *Psychiatry Research* 170, no. 1 (2009): 22–31.

59 Bernardo Dell'Osso, A. Carlo Altamura, Andrea Allen, Donatella Marazziti, and Eric Hollander, "Epidemiologic and clinical updates on impulse control disorders: A critical review," *European Archives of Psychiatry and Clinical Neuroscience* 256 (2006): 464–75.

60 Marc N. Potenza, Lorrin M. Koran, and Stefano Pallanti, "The relationship between impulse-control disorders and obsessive-compulsive disorder: A current understanding and future research directions," *Psychiatry Research* 170, no. 1 (2009): 22–31.

61 Ibid.

62 Jon E. Grant, Laura Levine, Daniel Kim, and Marc N. Potenza, "Impulse control disorders in adult psychiatric inpatients," *American Journal of Psychiatry* 162, no. 11 (2005): 2184–88.

63 O. Joseph Bienvenu, Jack F. Samuels, Mark A. Riddle, Rudolf Hoehn-Saric, Kung-Yee Liang, Bernadette A. M. Cullen, Marco A. Grados, and Gerald Nestadt, "The relationship of obsessive-compulsive disorder to possible spectrum disorders: Results from a family study," *Biological Psychiatry* 48 (2000): 287–93.

64 American Psychiatric Association, "*DSM-5 Development.*" http://www.dsm5.org/ProposedRevision/Pages/proposedrevision.aspx?rid=372# (accessed September 21, 2012).

65 Ibid.

66 Stephen A. Wonderlich, Kathryn H. Gordon, James E. Mitchell, Ross D. Crosby, and Scott G. Engel, "The validity and clinical utility of binge eating disorder," *International Journal of Eating Disorders* 42, no. 8 (2009): 687–705.

67 American Psychiatric Association, "*DSM–5 Development.*" http://www.dsm5.org/proposedrevision/Pages/FeedingandEatingDisorders.aspx (accessed September 21, 2012).

68 American Psychiatric Association, "*DSM–5 Development.*" http://www.dsm5.org/proposedrevision/Pages/NeurodevelopmentalDisorders.aspx (accessed September 25, 2012).

69 American Psychiatric Association, "*DSM–5 Development.*" http://www.dsm5.org/proposedrevision/Pages/FeedingandEatingDisorders.aspx (accessed September 25, 2012).

70 American Psychiatric Association, "*DSM–5 Development.*" http://www.dsm5.org/proposedrevision/Pages/Disruptive,ImpulseControl,andConductDisorders.aspx (accessed September 25, 2012).

71 American Psychiatric Association, "*DSM–5 Development.*" http://www.dsm5.org/ProposedRevision/Pages/proposedrevision.aspx?rid=71 (accessed September 25, 2012).

72 American Psychiatric Association, "*DSM–5 Development.*" http://www.dsm5.org/proposedrevision/Pages/SexualDysfunctions.aspx (accessed September 25, 2012).

73 American Psychiatric Association, "*DSM–5 Development.*" http://www.dsm5.org/proposedrevision/Pages/SubstanceUseandAddictiveDisorders.aspx (accessed September 25, 2012).

74 Jon E. Grant, *Impulse Control Disorders: A Clinician's Guide to Understanding and Treating Behavioral Addictions* (New York: W. W. Norton & Company, 2008).

75 Ronald C. Kessler and Philip S. Wang, "The descriptive epidemiology of commonly occurring mental disorders in the United States," *Annual Review of Public Health* 29 (2008): 115–29.

76 Ibid.

77 Jon E. Grant, Laura Levine, Daniel Kim, and Marc N. Potenza, "Impulse control disorders in adult psychiatric inpatients," *American Journal of Psychiatry* 162, no. 11 (2005): 2184–88.

78 Astrid Müller, Katharina Rein, Ines Kollei, Andrea Jacobi, Andrea Rotter, Patricia Schütz, Thomas Hillemacher, Martina de Zwaan, "Impulse control disorders in psychiatric inpatients," *Psychiatry Research* 188 (2011): 434–38.

79 Nancy M. Petry, "Should the scope of addictive behaviors be broadened to include pathological gambling?" *Addiction* 101, Suppl. 1 (2006): 152–60.

80 Aviv Weinstein and Michel Lejoyeux, "Internet addiction or excessive

Internet use," *The American Journal of Drug and Alcohol Abuse* 36 (2010): 277–83.

81 Frederico Garcia and Florence Thibaut, "Sexual addictions," *The American Journal of Drug and Alcohol Abuse* 36 (2010): 254–60.

82 L. E. Marshall and W. L. Marshall, "Sexual addiction in incarcerated sexual offenders," *Sexual Addiction & Compulsivity* 13 (2006): 377–90.

83 Lorrin M. Koran, Ronald J. Faber, Elias Aboujaoude, Michael D. Large, and Richard T. Serpe, "Estimated prevalence of compulsive buying behavior in the United States," *The American Journal of Psychiatry* 163 (2006): 1806–12.

84 Michel Lejoyeux and Aviv Weinstein, "Compulsive buying," *The American Journal of Drug and Alcohol Abuse* 36 (2010): 248–53.

85 James Hudson, Eva Hiripi, Harrison Pope, Jr., and Ronald Kessler, "The prevalence and correlates of eating disorders in the National Comorbidity Survey Replication," *Biological Psychiatry* 61 (2007): 348–58.

86 Susan Z. Yanovski, "Binge eating disorder and obesity in 2003: Could treating an eating disorder have a positive effect on the obesity epidemic?" *International Journal of Eating Disorders* 34 (2003): 117–20.

87 M. de Zwaan, "Binge eating disorder and obesity," *International Journal of Obesity* 25, Suppl. 1 (2001): 51–55.

88 Substance Abuse and Mental Health Services Administration, "Results from the 2010 National Survey on Drug Use and Health: Summary of National Findings," NSDUH Series H-41, HHS Publication No. (SMA) 11-4658 (Rockville, MD: Substance Abuse and Mental Health Services Administration, 2011).

89 Jon E. Grant, *Impulse Control Disorders: A Clinician's Guide to Understanding and Treating Behavioral Addictions* (New York: W. W. Norton & Company, 2008).

90 Ibid.

91 Nora D. Volkow, Joanna S. Fowler, and Gene-Jack Wang, "The addicted human brain viewed in the light of imaging studies: Brain circuits and treatment strategies," *Neuropharmacology*, Supplement 1, vol. 47 (2004): 3–13.

92 Isaac Marks, "Editorial: Behavioural (non-chemical) addictions," *British Journal of Addiction* 85, no. 11 (1990): 1389.

93 Peter R. Martin and Nancy Petry, "Are non-substance-related addictions really addictions?" *The American Journal on Addictions* 14 (2005): 2.

94 National Institute on Drug Abuse, "Drugs, brains, and behavior: The science of addiction" (2010), http://www.drugabuse.gov/sites/default/files/sciofaddiction.pdf (accessed October 19, 2012).

95 Ulrike Albrecht, Nina E. Kirschner, and Sabine M. Grüsser, "Diagnostic instruments for behavioral addiction: An overview," *GMS Psycho-Social-Medicine* 4, doc. 11 (2007): 1–11.

96 Peter R. Martin and Nancy Petry, "Are non-substance-related addictions really addictions?" *The American Journal on Addictions* 14 (2005): 2.

97 Christopher M. Olsen, "Natural rewards, neuroplasticity, and non-drug addictions," *Neuropharmacology* 61, no. 7 (2011): 1109–10.

98 Joseph Frascella, Marc N. Potenza, Lucy L. Brown, and Anna Rose Childress, "Shared brain vulnerabilities open the way for nonsubstance addictions: Carving addiction at a new joint?" *Annals of the New York Academy of Sciences*, Addiction Reviews 2, vol. 1187 (2010): 294–315.

99 Shirley Lee, and Avis Mysyk, "The medicalization of compulsive buying," *Social Science & Medicine* 58, no. 9 (2004): 1709–18.

100 Ibid.

101 Ibid. 1713

102 Ibid.

103 Kimberly S. Young, "Internet sex addiction: Risk factors, stages of development, and treatment," *American Behavioral Scientist* 52, no. 1 (2008): 21–37.

104 Ibid. 22

105 Nora D. Volkow and Roy A. Wise, "How can drug addiction help us understand obesity?" *Nature Neuroscience* 8 (2005): 555.

106 Ibid.

107 Nancy M. Petry, Frederick S. Stinson, and Bridget F. Grant, "Comorbidity of DSM-IV pathological gambling and other psychiatric disorders: Results from the National Epidemiologic Survey on Alcohol and Related Conditions," *Journal of Clinical Psychiatry* 66, no. 5 (2005): 564–74.

108 Marco Di Nicola, Daniela Tedeschi, Marianna Mazza, Giovanni Martinotti, Desiree Harnic, Valeria Catalano, Angelo Bruschi, Gino Pozzi, Pietro Bria, and Luigi Janiri, "Behavioral addictions in bipolar disorder patients: Role of impulsivity and personality dimensions," *Journal of Affective Disorder* 125 (2010): 82–88.

109 Ju-Yu Yen, Chih-Hung Ko, Chen-Fang Yen, Sue-Huei Chen, Wei-Lun Chung, and Cheng-Chung Chen, "Psychiatric symptoms in adolescents with Internet addiction: Comparison with substance use," *Psychiatry and Clinical Neurosciences* 62, no. 1 (2008): 9–16.

110 Center for Substance Abuse Treatment, *Substance Abuse Treatment for Persons with Co-Occurring Disorders*, Treatment Improvement Protocol (TIP) Series 42, DHHS Publication No. (SMA) 08-3992 (Rockville, MD: Substance Abuse and Mental Health Services Administration, 2005).

111 Ju-Yu Yen, Chih-Hung Ko, Chen-Fang Yen, Sue-Huei Chen, Wei-Lun Chung, and Cheng-Chung Chen, "Psychiatric symptoms in adolescents with Internet addiction: Comparison with substance use," *Psychiatry and Clinical Neurosciences* 62, no. 1 (2008): 9–16.

112 Peter R. Martin and Nancy Petry, "Are non-substance-related addictions really addictions?" *The American Journal on Addictions* 14 (2005): 2.

CHAPTER TWO

1 American Psychiatric Association, *Diagnostic and Statistical Manual of Mental Disorders, Fourth Edition, Text Revision* (Washington, DC: American Psychiatric Publishing, 2000).

2 Robin A. Hurley, Ronald E. Fisher, and Katherine H. Taber, "Clinical and Functional Imaging in Neuropsychiatry," in *Essentials of Neuropsychiatry and Behavioral Neurosciences* (Second Edition), ed. by Stuart C. Yudofsky and Robert E. Hales (Washington DC: American Psychiatric Publishing Inc., 2010), 55–94.

3 Carlton K. Erickson, *The Science of Addiction: From Neurobiology to Treatment* (New York: W. W. Norton & Company, 2007), 33–39.

4 A. Kimberly McAllister, W. Martin Usrey, Stephen C. Noctor, and Stephen Rayport, "Fundamentals of Cellular Neurobiology," in *Essentials of Neuropsychiatry and Behavioral Neurosciences,* ed. by Stuart C. Yudofsky and Robert E. Hales (Washington DC: American Psychiatric Publishing Inc., 2010), 1–28.

5 Ibid.

6 Ibid.

7 Eric J. Nestler and David W. Self, "Neuropsychiatric Aspects of Ethanol

and Other Chemical Dependencies," in *Essentials of Neuropsychiatry and Behavioral Neurosciences,* ed. by Stuart C. Yudofsky and Robert E. Hales (Washington DC: American Psychiatric Publishing Inc., 2010), 369–86.

8 A. Kimberly McAllister, W. Martin Usrey, Stephen C. Noctor, and Stephen Rayport, "Fundamentals of Cellular Neurobiology," in *Essentials of Neuropsychiatry and Behavioral Neurosciences,* ed. by Stuart C. Yudofsky and Robert E. Hales (Washington DC: American Psychiatric Publishing Inc., 2010), 1–28.

9 Ibid.

10 Carlton K. Erickson, *The Science of Addiction: From Neurobiology to Treatment* (New York: W. W. Norton & Company, 2007), 39.

11 Ibid.

12 George F. Koob and Michel Le Moal, *Neurobiology of Addiction* (London: Elsevier, 2006), 447–48.

13 Carlton K. Erickson, *The Science of Addiction: From Neurobiology to Treatment* (New York: W. W. Norton & Company, 2007), 50–73.

14 Marc N. Potenza, "The neurobiology of pathological gambling and drug addiction: an overview and new findings," *Philosophical Transactions of the Royal Society B (Biological Sciences)* 363 (2008): 3181–89.

15 Carlton K. Erickson, *The Science of Addiction: From Neurobiology to Treatment* (New York: W. W. Norton & Company, 2007), 50–73.

16 Ibid.

17 A. Kimberly McAllister, W. Martin Usrey, Stephen C. Noctor, and Stephen Rayport, "Fundamentals of Cellular Neurobiology," in *Essentials of Neuropsychiatry and Behavioral Neurosciences,* ed. by Stuart C. Yudofsky and Robert E. Hales (Washington DC: American Psychiatric Publishing Inc., 2010), 1–28.

18 Eric J. Nestler and David W. Self, "Neuropsychiatric Aspects of Ethanol and Other Chemical Dependencies," in *Essentials of Neuropsychiatry and Behavioral Neurosciences,* ed. by Stuart C. Yudofsky and Robert E. Hales (Washington DC: American Psychiatric Publishing Inc., 2010), 369–86.

19 Peter W. Kalivas and Nora D. Volkow, "The neural basis of addiction: A pathology of motivation and choice, *American Journal of Psychiatry* 162, no. 8 (2005): 1403–13.

20 Barry J. Everitt and Trevor W. Robbins, "Neural systems of reinforcement for drug addiction: From actions to habits to compulsion," *Nature Neuroscience* 8 (2005): 1481–89.

21 Roy A. Wise, "Action of drugs of abuse on brain reward systems," *Pharmacology Biochemistry and Behavior* 13, supp. 1 (1980): 213–23.

22 Roy A. Wise, "Brain reward circuitry: insights from unsensed incentives," *Neuron* 36 (2002): 229–40.

CHAPTER THREE

1 Nancy M. Petry, *Pathological Gambling: Etiology, Comorbidity, and Treatment* (Washington DC: American Psychological Association, 2005), 4.

2 David M. Haugen, *Legalized Gambling (*New York, NY: Infobase Publishing, 2006).

3 Nancy M. Petry, *Pathological Gambling: Etiology, Comorbidity, and Treatment* (Washington DC: American Psychological Association, 2005).

4 Rod L. Evans and Mark Hance, *Legalized Gambling: For and Against* (Chicago, IL: Open Court Publishing Company, 1998).

5 Paul Ruschmann, *Legalized Gambling* (New York, NY: Chelsea House Publishers, 2009).

6 National Gambling Impact Study Commission (NGISC), *Final Report* (Washington DC: Government Printing Office, 1999).

7 R. Keith Schwer, William N. Thompson, and Daryl Nakamuro, "Beyond the limits of recreation: Social costs of gambling in Southern Nevada." Paper presented at the annual meeting of the Far West and American Popular Culture Association, Las Vegas, NV, February 1, 2003.

8 National Research Council (NRC), *Pathological Gambling: A Critical Review* (Washington DC: National Academy Press, 1999).

9 Nancy M. Petry, *Pathological Gambling: Etiology, Comorbidity, and Treatment* (Washington DC: American Psychological Association, 2005).

10 John W. Kindt, "The failure to regulate the gambling industry effectively: Incentives for perpetual non-compliance," *Southern Illinois University Law Journal* 27 (2002): 221–62.

11 Marc N. Potenza, "The neurobiology of pathological gambling and drug addiction: An overview and new findings," *Philosophical Transactions of The Royal Society B (Biological Sciences)* 363 (2008): 3181–89.

12 Howard J. Shaffer and David A. Korn, "Gambling and related mental disorders: A public health analysis," *Annual Review of Public Health* 23 (2002): 171–212.

13 Tian P. S. Oei and Leon M. Gordon, "Psychosocial factors related to gambling abstinence and relapse in members of Gamblers Anonymous," *Journal of Gambling Studies* 24, no. 1 (2008): 91–105.

14 Marc N. Potenza, "The neurobiology of pathological gambling and drug addiction: An overview and new findings," *Philosophical Transactions of The Royal Society B (Biological Sciences)* 363 (2008): 2181–89.

15 Harvard Health Publications, "Pathological gambling," *Harvard Mental Health Letter* (August 2010) (Boston, MA: Harvard Health Publications, Harvard Medical School Harvard University, 2010).

16 Jon E. Grant, Marc N. Potenza, Aviv Weinstein, and David A. Gorelick, "Introduction to behavioral addictions," *The American Journal of Drug and Alcohol Abuse* 36, no. 5 (September 2010): 233–41.

17 Denise Phillips, "Gambling: The hidden addiction: cases of this psychiatric disorder are on the rise as more Americans fall under the spell of 'Lady Luck' (Addictions)," *Behavioral Health Management* 25, no. 5 (September 2005): 32–37.

18 Nancy M. Petry, *Pathological Gambling: Etiology, Comorbidity, and Treatment* (Washington DC: American Psychological Association, 2005).

19 Wendy S. Slutske, "Natural recovery and treatment-seeking in pathological gambling: Results of two US national surveys," *American Journal of Psychiatry* 163, no. 2 (2006): 297–302.

20 Howard J. Shaffer, Matthew N. Hall, and Joni Vander Bilt, "Estimating the prevalence of disordered gambling behavior in the United States and Canada: A research synthesis. *American Journal of Public Health,* 89 (1999): 1369–76.

21 Robert L. Custer and Harry Milt, *When Luck Runs Out: Help for Compulsive Gamblers and Their Families* (New York: Facts on File, 1985).

22 Nancy M. Petry, *Pathological Gambling: Etiology, Comorbidity, and Treatment* (Washington DC: American Psychological Association, 2005).

23 Ibid.

24 Denise Phillips, "Gambling: The hidden addiction: cases of this psychiatric disorder are on the rise as more Americans fall under the spell of 'Lady Luck' (Addictions)," *Behavioral Health Management* 25, no. 5 (September 2005): 32–37.

25 Robert L. Custer and Harry Milt, *When Luck Runs Out: Help for Compulsive Gamblers and Their Families* (New York: Facts on File, 1985).

26 Denise Phillips, "Gambling: The hidden addiction: cases of this psychiatric disorder are on the rise as more Americans fall under the spell of 'Lady Luck.' (Addictions)," *Behavioral Health Management* 25, no. 5 (September 2005): 32–37.

27 Nigel E. Turner, Umesh Jain, Warren Spence, and Masood Zangeneh, "Pathways to pathological gambling: Component analysis of variables related to pathological gambling," *International Gambling Studies* 8, no. 3 (2008): 281–98.

28 Louise Sharpe, "A reformulated cognitive-behavioral model of problem gambling: A biopsychosocial perspective," *Clinical Psychology Review* 22, no. 1 (2002): 1–25.

29 Rina Gupta and Jeffrey L. Derevensky, "A treatment approach for adolescents with gambling problems," in *Gambling Problems in Youth: Theoretical and Applied Perspectives*, ed. by Jeffrey Derevensky and Rina Gupta (New York: Kluwer Academic/Plenum Publishers, 2004), 165–88.

30 Lia Nower and Alex Blaszczynski, "A pathways approach to treating youth gamblers," in *Gambling Problems in Youth: Theoretical and Applied Perspectives*, ed. by Jeffrey L. Derevensky and Rina Gupta (New York: Kluwer Academic/Plenum Publishers, 2004), 189–209.

31 Nigel E. Turner, Umesh Jain, Warren Spence, and Masood Zangeneh, "Pathways to pathological gambling: Component analysis of variables related to pathological gambling," *International Gambling Studies* 8, no. 3 (2008): 281–98.

32 Alex Blaszczynski and Eimear Farrell, "A case series of 44 completed gambling-related suicides," *Journal of Gambling Studies* 14, no. 2 (1998): 93–109.

33 Lia Nower and Alex Blaszczynski, "Recovery in pathological gambling: An imprecise concept," *Substance Use and Misuse* 43, no. 12–13 (2008): 1844–64.

34 Ibid.

35 Lia Nower and Alex Blaszczynski, "A pathways approach to treating youth gamblers," in *Gambling Problems in Youth: Theoretical and Applied Perspectives*, ed. by Jeffrey L. Derevensky and Rina Gupta (New York: Kluwer Academic/Plenum Publishers, 2004), 189–209.

36 Lia Nower and Alex Blaszczynski, "Recovery in pathological gambling: An imprecise concept," *Substance Use and Misuse* 43, no. 12–13 (2008): 1844–64.

37 Howard J. Shaffer and David A. Korn, "Gambling and related mental disorders: A public health analysis," *Annual Review of Public Health* 23 (2002): 171–212.

38 Jochen Mutschler, Mira Bühler, Martin Grosshans, Alexander Diehl, Karl Mann, and Falk Kiefer, "Disulfiram, an option for the treatment of pathological gambling?" *Alcohol and Alcoholism* 45, no. 2 (2010): 214–16.

39 Howard J. Shaffer, Debi A. LaPlante, Richard A. LaBrie, Rachel C. Kidman, Anthony N. Donato, and Michael V. Stanton, "Toward a syndrome model of addiction: Multiple expressions, common etiology," *Harvard Review of Psychiatry* 12 (2004): 367–74.

40 Jeffrey L. Derevensky and Rina Gupta, *Gambling Problems in Youth: Theoretical and Applied Perspectives* (New York: Kluwer Academic/Plenum Publishers, 2004).

41 Carlos Blanco, Angela Ibáñez, Jerónimo Sáiz-Ruiz, Carmen Blanco-Jerez, and Edward V. Nunes, "Epidemiology, pathophysiology and treatment of pathological gambling," *CNS Drugs* 13, no. 6 (June 2000): 397–407.

42 Iulian Iancu, Katherine Lowengrub, Yael Dembinsky, Moshe Kotler, and Pinhas N. Dannon, "Pathological Gambling: An update on neuropathophysiology and pharmacotherapy," *CNS Drugs* 22, no. 2 (2008): 123–38.

43 Ibid.

44 Ibid.

45 Jeffrey L. Derevensky and Rina Gupta, *Gambling Problems in Youth: Theoretical and Applied Perspectives* (New York: Kluwer Academic/Plenum Publishers, 2004).

46 Ibid.

47 Stephen R. McDaniel and Marvin Zuckerman, "The relationship of impulsive sensation seeking and gender to interest and participation in gambling activities," *Personality and Individual Differences* 35, no. 6 (October 2003): 1385–1400.

48 Jeffrey L. Derevensky and Rina Gupta, *Gambling Problems in Youth: Theoretical and Applied Perspectives* (New York: Kluwer Academic/Plenum Publishers, 2004).

49 Owen Richard Lightsey, Jr. and C. Duncan Hulsey, "Impulsivity, coping, stress, and problem gambling among university students," *Journal of Counseling Psychology* 49, no. 2 (April 2002): 202–11.

50 Jeffrey L. Derevensky and Rina Gupta, *Gambling Problems in Youth: Theoretical and Applied Perspectives* (New York: Kluwer Academic/Plenum Publishers, 2004).

51 Henry R. Lesieur and Sheila Blume, "When Lady Luck loses: Women and Compulsive Gambling" in *Feminist Perspective on Addictions,* ed. by Nan Van Den Bergh (New York: Springer, 1991), 181–97.

52 Otto Kausch, Loreen Rugle, and Douglas Y. Rowland, "Lifetime histories of trauma among pathological gamblers," *The American Journal on Addictions* 15, no. 1 (January-February 2006): 35–43.

53 Patrick B. Johnson and Micheline S. Malow-Iroff, *Adolescents and Risk: Making Sense of Adolescent Psychology. Making Sense of Psychology*, Carol Korn-Bursztyn, Series Editor (Westport, CT: Praeger Publishers, 2008), 40.

54 Agneta Johansson, Jon E. Grant, Suck Won Kim, Brian L. Odlaug, and K. Gunnar Götestam, "Risk factors for problematic gambling: A critical literature review," *Journal of Gambling Studies* 25 (2009): 67–92.

55 Iulian Iancu, Katherine Lowengrub, Yael Dembinsky, Moshe Kotler, and Pinhas N. Dannon, "Pathological Gambling: An update on neuropathophysiology and pharmacotherapy," *CNS Drugs* 22, no. 2 (2008): 123–38.

56 Carlos Blanco, Angela Ibáñez, Jerónimo Sáiz-Ruiz, Carmen Blanco-Jerez, and Edward V. Nunes, "Epidemiology, pathophysiology and treatment of pathological gambling," *CNS Drugs* 13, no. 6 (June 2000): 397–407.

57 Dean Gerstein, Sally Murphy, Marianna Toce, John Hoffman, Amanda Palmer, Robert Johnson, Cindy Larison, Lucian Chuchro, Tracy Buie, Laszlo Engelman, and Mary A. Hill, *Gambling Impact and Behavior Study: Report to the National Gambling Impact Study Commission* (Chicago: National Opinion Research Center at the University of Chicago, 1999).

58 Howard J. Shaffer and David A. Korn, "Gambling and related mental disorders: A public health analysis," *Annual Review of Public Health* 23 (2002): 171–212.

59 Nancy M. Petry, *Pathological Gambling: Etiology, Comorbidity, and Treatment* (Washington DC: American Psychological Association, 2005).

60 Denise Phillips, "Gambling: The hidden addiction: cases of this psychiatric

disorder are on the rise as more Americans fall under the spell of 'Lady Luck' (Addictions)," *Behavioral Health Management* 25, no. 5 (September 2005): 32–37.

61 Otto Kausch, "Patterns of substance abuse among treatment-seeking pathological gamblers," *Journal of Substance Abuse Treatment* 25, no. 4 (December 2003): 263–70.

62 Denise Phillips, "Gambling: The hidden addiction: cases of this psychiatric disorder are on the rise as more Americans fall under the spell of 'Lady Luck' (Addictions)," *Behavioral Health Management* 25, no. 5 (September 2005): 32–37.

63 Otto Kausch, "Patterns of substance abuse among treatment-seeking pathological gamblers," *Journal of Substance Abuse Treatment* 25, no. 4 (December 2003): 263–70.

64 Denise Phillips, "Gambling: The hidden addiction: cases of this psychiatric disorder are on the rise as more Americans fall under the spell of 'Lady Luck' (Addictions)," *Behavioral Health Management* 25 no. 5 (September 2005): 32–37.

65 Nancy M. Petry, *Pathological Gambling: Etiology, Comorbidity, and Treatment* (Washington DC: American Psychological Association, 2005).

66 Denise Phillips, "Gambling: The hidden addiction: cases of this psychiatric disorder are on the rise as more Americans fall under the spell of 'Lady Luck' (Addictions)," *Behavioral Health Management* 25, no. 5 (September 2005): 32–37.

67 Ibid.

68 Howard J. Shaffer and David A. Korn, "Gambling and related mental disorders: A public health analysis," *Annual Review of Public Health* 23 (2002): 171–212.

69 Nancy M. Petry, *Pathological Gambling: Etiology, Comorbidity, and Treatment* (Washington DC: American Psychological Association, 2005).

70 Alex Blaszczynski and Eimear Farrell, "A case series of 44 completed gambling-related suicides," *Journal of Gambling Studies* 14, no. 2 (1998): 93–109.

71 Lia Nower, "Pathological gamblers in the workplace: A primer for employers," *Employee Assistance Quarterly* 18, no. 4 (2003): 55–72.

72 John W. Kindt, "The failure to regulate the gambling industry effectively: Incentives for perpetual non-compliance," *Southern Illinois University Law Journal* 27 (2002): 221–62.

73 Howard J. Shaffer and David A. Korn, "Gambling and related mental disorders: A public health analysis," *Annual Review of Public Health* 23 (2002): 171–212.

74 Lia Nower, "Pathological gamblers in the workplace: A primer for employers," *Employee Assistance Quarterly* 18, no. 4 (2003): 55–72.

75 Michel Lejoyeux, Nathalie Feuché, Sabrina Loi, Jacquelyn Solomon, and Jean Adès, "Study of impulsive-control disorders among alcohol-dependent patients," *Journal of Clinical Psychiatry* 60 (1999): 302–05.

76 Robert D. Linden, Harrison G. Pope, and Jeffrey M. Jonas, "Pathological gambling and major affective disorder: Preliminary findings," *Journal of Clinical Psychiatry* 47, no. 4 (1986): 201–03.

77 R. Keith Schwer, William N. Thompson, and Daryl Nakamuro, "Beyond the limits of recreation: Social costs of gambling in Southern Nevada." Paper presented at the annual meeting of the Far West and American Popular Culture Association, Las Vegas, NV, February 1, 2003.

78 David N. Crockford and Nady el-Guebaly, "Psychiatric comorbidity in pathological gambling: A critical review," *Canadian Journal of Psychiatry* 43, no. 1 (1998): 43–50.

79 David C. Hodgins, Chrystal Mansley, and Kylie Thygesen, "Risk factors for suicide ideation and attempts among pathological gamblers," *The American Journal of Addictions* 15, no. 4 (2006): 303–10.

80 Ibid.

81 Nancy M. Petry, *Pathological Gambling: Etiology, Comorbidity, and Treatment* (Washington DC: American Psychological Association, 2005).

82 Rachel A. Volberg, "The prevalence and demographics of pathological gamblers: Implications for public health," *American Journal of Public Health* 84, no. 2 (February 1994): 217–41.

83 Jon E. Grant, Marc N. Potenza, Aviv Weinstein, and David A. Gorelick, "Introduction to behavioral addictions," *The American Journal of Drug and Alcohol Abuse* 36, no. 5 (September 2010): 233–41.

84 George T. Ladd and Nancy M. Petry, "Gender differences among pathological gamblers seeking treatment," *Experimental and Clinical Psychopharmacology* 10, no. 3 (August 2002): 302–09.

85 Nigel E. Turner, Umesh Jain, Warren Spence, and Masood Zangeneh, "Pathways to pathological gambling: Component analysis of variables related to pathological gambling," *International Gambling Studies* 8, no. 3 (2008): 281–98.

86 Roberta Boughton and Olesya Falenchuk, "Vulnerability and comorbidity factors of female problem gambling," *Journal of Gambling Studies* 23, no. 3 (2007): 323–34.

87 Durand F. Jacobs, "Youth gambling in North America: Long-term trends and future prospects," in *Gambling Problems in Youth: Theoretical and Applied Perspectives*, ed. by Jeffrey L. Derevensky and Rina Gupta (New York: Kluwer Academic/Plenum Publishers, 2004), 1–26.

88 Ibid.

89 Jeffrey L. Derevensky and Rina Gupta, *Gambling Problems in Youth: Theoretical and Applied Perspectives* (New York: Kluwer Academic/Plenum Publishers, 2004).

90 Howard J. Shaffer and David A. Korn, "Gambling and related mental disorders: A public health analysis," *Annual Review of Public Health* 23 (2002): 171–212.

91 Rani A. Desai, Paul K. Maciejewski, David J. Dausey, Barbara J. Caldarone, and Marc N. Potenza, "Health correlates of recreational gambling in older adults," *American Journal of Psychiatry* 161, no. 9 (2004): 1672–79.

92 Illinois Department on Aging, "Action vs. escape gamblers," Illinois Department on Aging, 2005. http://www.state.il.us/aging/3hot/gambling_act-esc.htm (accessed June 11, 2012).

93 Denise Phillips, "Gambling: The hidden addiction: cases of this psychiatric disorder are on the rise as more Americans fall under the spell of 'Lady Luck' (Addictions)," *Behavioral Health Management* 25, no. 5 (September 2005): 32–37.

94 William George McCown and Linda L. Chamberlain, *Best Possible Odds: Contemporary Treatment Strategies for Gambling Disorders* (New York: John Wiley & Sons, 2000).

95 Nancy M. Petry, *Pathological Gambling: Etiology, Comorbidity, and Treatment* (Washington DC: American Psychological Association, 2005).

96 Denise Phillips, "Gambling: The hidden addiction: cases of this psychiatric disorder are on the rise as more Americans fall under the spell of 'Lady Luck' (Addictions)," *Behavioral Health Management* 25, no. 5 (September 2005): 32–37.

97 Nancy M. Petry, *Pathological Gambling: Etiology, Comorbidity, and Treatment* (Washington DC: American Psychological Association, 2005).

98 Joseph W. Ciarrocchi, *Counseling Problem Gamblers: A Self-Regulation Manual for Individual and Family Therapy* (San Diego: Academic Press, 2002).

99 Denise Phillips, "Gambling: The hidden addiction: cases of this psychiatric disorder are on the rise as more Americans fall under the spell of 'Lady Luck' (Addictions)," *Behavioral Health Management* 25, no. 5 (September 2005): 32–37.

100 John A. Cunningham, "Little use of treatment among problem gamblers," *Psychiatric Services* 56, no. 8 (2005): 1024–25.

101 Wendy S. Slutske, "Natural recovery and treatment-seeking in pathological gambling: Results of two U.S. national surveys," *American Journal of Psychiatry* 163, no. 2 (2006): 297–302.

102 Helen Suurvali, David C. Hodgins, and John A. Cunningham, "Motivators for resolving or seeking help for gambling problems: A review of the empirical literature," *Journal of Gambling Studies* 26 (2010): 1–33.

103 Ibid.

104 Tony Toneatto and Robert Ladoceur, "The treatment of pathological gambling: A critical review of the literature," *Psychology of Addictive Behaviors* 17 (2003): 284–92.

105 Damon Lipinski, James P. Whelan, and Andrew W. Meyers, "Treatment of pathological gambling using a guided self-change approach," *Clinical Case Studies* 6, no. 5 (October 2007): 394–411.

106 Jon E. Grant, Marc N. Potenza, Aviv Weinstein, and David A. Gorelick, "Introduction to behavioral addictions," *The American Journal of Drug and Alcohol Abuse* 36, no. 5 (September 2010): 233–41.

107 Patrick B. Johnson and Micheline S. Malow-Iroff, *Adolescents and Risk: Making Sense of Adolescent Psychology. Making Sense of Psychology*, Carol Korn-Bursztyn, Series Editor (Westport, CT: Praeger Publishers, 2008).

108 Gerald Corey, *Theory and Practice of Counseling and Psychotherapy, Seventh Edition* (Belmont, CA: Brooks/Cole-Thompson Learning, 2005).

109 Robert Ladouceur and Michael B. Walker, "Cognitive approach to understanding and treating pathological gambling," in *Comprehensive Clinical Psychology*, ed. by Allen S. Bellack and Michel Hersen (New York: Pergamon, 1998), 587–601.

110 Rina Gupta and Jeffrey L. Derevensky, "A treatment approach for adolescents with gambling problems," in *Gambling Problems in Youth: Theoretical and Applied Perspectives*, ed. by Jeffrey Derevensky and Rina Gupta (New York: Kluwer Academic/Plenum Publishers, 2004), 165–88.

111 Nancy M. Petry, Mark D. Litt, Ronald Kadden, and David M. Ledgerwood, "Do coping skills mediate the relationship between cognitive-behavioral therapy and reductions in gambling in pathological gamblers?" *Addiction* 102, no. 8 (2007): 1280–91.

112 Iulian Iancu, Katherine Lowengrub, Yael Dembinsky, Moshe Kotler, and Pinhas N. Dannon, "Pathological Gambling: An update on neuropathophysiology and pharmacotherapy," *CNS Drugs* 22, no. 2 (2008): 123–38.

113 Robert Ladouceur and Stella LaChance, *Overcoming Pathological Gambling: A Therapist Guide* (New York: Oxford University Press, 2007).

114 Damon Lipinski, James P. Whelan, and Andrew W. Meyers, "Treatment of pathological gambling using a guided self-change approach," *Clinical Case Studies* 6, no. 5 (October 2007): 394–411.

115 Robert Ladouceur and Stella LaChance, *Overcoming Pathological Gambling: A Therapist Guide* (New York: Oxford University Press, 2007).

116 Damon Lipinski, James P. Whelan, and Andrew W. Meyers, "Treatment of pathological gambling using a guided self-change approach," *Clinical Case Studies* 6, no. 5 (October 2007): 394–411.

117 Robert Ladouceur, Caroline Sylvain, Claude Boutin, and Celine Doucet, *Understanding and Treating the Pathological Gambler* (West Sussex: John Wiley & Sons, Inc., 2003).

118 Robert Ladouceur and Stella LaChance, *Overcoming Pathological Gambling: A Therapist Guide* (New York: Oxford University Press, 2007).

119 Helen Suurvali, David C. Hodgins, and John A. Cunningham, "Motivators for resolving or seeking help for gambling problems: A review of the empirical literature," *Journal of Gambling Studies* 26 (2010): 1–33.

120 Wendy S. Slutske, "Natural recovery and treatment-seeking in pathological gambling: Results of two U.S. national surveys," *American Journal of Psychiatry*, 163, no. 2 (2006): 297–302.

121 Jochen Mutschler, Mira Bühler, Martin Grosshans, Alexander Diehl, Karl Mann, and Falk Kiefer, "Disulfiram, an option for the treatment of pathological gambling?" *Alcohol and Alcoholism* 45, no. 2 (2010): 214–16.

122 Jon E. Grant, Marc N. Potenza, Aviv Weinstein, and David A. Gorelick, "Introduction to behavioral addictions," *The American Journal of Drug and Alcohol Abuse* 36, no. 5 (September 2010): 233–41.

123 Jochen Mutschler, Mira Bühler, Martin Grosshans, Alexander Diehl, Karl Mann, and Falk Kiefer, "Disulfiram, an option for the treatment of pathological gambling?" *Alcohol and Alcoholism* 45, no. 2 (2010): 214–16.

124 Nancy M. Petry, *Pathological Gambling: Etiology, Comorbidity, and Treatment* (Washington DC: American Psychological Association, 2005).

125 Ibid.

126 Ibid.

127 Howard J. Shaffer and David A. Korn, "Gambling and related mental disorders: A public health analysis," *Annual Review of Public Health* 23 (2002): 171–212.

128 Jeffrey L. Derevensky, Rina Gupta, Laurie Dickson, and Anne-Elyse Deguire, "Prevention efforts toward reducing gambling problems," in *Gambling Problems in Youth: Theoretical and Applied Perspectives*, ed. by Jeffrey L. Derevensky and Rina Gupta (New York: Kluwer Academic/Plenum Publishers, 2004), 211–30.

129 Ibid.

130 Howard J. Shaffer and David A. Korn, "Gambling and related mental disorders: A public health analysis," *Annual Review of Public Health* 23 (2002): 171–212.

CHAPTER FOUR

1 Marnie C. Ferree, "Females and sex addiction: Myths and diagnostic implications." *Sexual Addiction and Compulsivity*, volume 8, issue 3–4 (2001): 287–300.

2 Tiffany Lee and Angela Kent, "Sexual addiction: Screening, assessment, diagnostic criteria, and treatment options," Western Michigan University, 2010.

3 Kenneth M. Adams and Donald W. Robinson, "Shame reduction, affect regulation, and sexual boundary development: Essential building blocks of sexual addiction treatment," *Sexual Addiction & Compulsivity*, volume 8, issue 1 (2001): 23.

4 Ibid. 25.

5 Patrick Carnes, *Out of the Shadows: Understanding Sexual Addiction,* Center City, MN: Hazelden Information and Education, 2001.

6 Ibid.

7 Martin Plant and Moira Plant, "Sex addiction: A comparison with dependence on psychoactive drugs," *Journal of Substance Use*, volume 8, number 4 (2003): 262.

8 Ibid.

9 Kenneth M. Adams and Donald W. Robinson, "Shame reduction, affect regulation, and sexual boundary development: Essential building blocks of sexual addiction treatment," *Sexual Addiction & Compulsivity*, volume 8, issue 1 (2001): 24.

10 Martin Plant and Moira Plant, "Sex addiction: A comparison with dependence on psychoactive drugs," *Journal of Substance Use*, volume 8, number 4 (2003): 262.

11 Patrick J. Carnes, Robert E. Murray, Louis Charpenter, "Bargains with chaos: Sex addicts and addiction interaction disorder," *Sexual Addiction & Compulsivity*, volume 12 (2005): 80.

12 Cynthia Power, "Food and sex addiction: Helping the clinician recognize and treat the interaction," *Sexual Addiction & Compulsivity*, volume 12 (2005): 220.

13 Richard Blankenship and Mark Laaser, "Sexual addiction and ADHD: Is there a connection?," *Sexual Addiction & Compulsivity*, volume 11 (2004): 9.

14 Suaye Anna Maria Valenti, "Use of object relations and self-psychology as treatment for sex addiction with a female borderline patient," *Sexual Addiction & Compulsivity*, volume 9, issue 4 (2002): 249–62.

15 Jon E. Grant and Marvin A. Steinberg, "Compulsive sexual behavior and pathological gambling," *Sexual Addiction & Compulsivity*, volume 12 (2005): 235–44.

16 Patrick J. Carnes, Robert E. Murray, Louis Charpenter, "Bargains with chaos: Sex addicts and addiction interaction disorder," *Sexual Addiction & Compulsivity*, volume 12 (2005): 79–120.

17 Patrick J. Carnes, Robert E. Murray, Louis Charpenter, "Bargains with chaos: Sex addicts and addiction interaction disorder," *Sexual Addiction & Compulsivity*, volume 12 (2005): 98.

18 Suaye Anna Maria Valenti, "Use of object relations and self-psychology as treatment for sex addiction with a female borderline patient," *Sexual Addiction & Compulsivity*, volume 9, issue 4 (2002): 249–62.

19 Richard Leedes, "The three most important criteria in diagnosing sexual addictions: Obsession, obsession, and obsession," *Sexual Addiction & Compulsivity*, volume 8 (2001): 215–26.

20 Patrick J. Carnes, Robert E. Murray, Louis Charpenter, "Bargains with chaos: Sex addicts and addiction interaction disorder," *Sexual Addiction & Compulsivity*, volume 12 (2005): 79–120.

21 Kenneth M. Adams and Donald W. Robinson, "Shame reduction, affect regulation, and sexual boundary development: Essential building blocks of sexual addiction treatment," *Sexual Addiction & Compulsivity*, volume 8, issue 1 (2001): 25.

22 Ibid. 26.

23 Ibid. 26.

24 Ibid. 23.

25 Ibid. 25.

26 Richard Leedes, "The three most important criteria in diagnosing sexual addictions: Obsession, obsession, and obsession," *Sexual Addiction & Compulsivity*, volume 8 (2001): 220.

27 Suaye Anna Maria Valenti, "Use of object relations and self-psychology as treatment for sex addiction with a female borderline patient," *Sexual Addiction & Compulsivity*, volume 9, issue 4 (2002): 249–262.

28 Kenneth M. Adams and Donald W. Robinson, "Shame reduction, affect regulation, and sexual boundary development: Essential building blocks of sexual addiction treatment," *Sexual Addiction & Compulsivity*, volume 8, issue 1 (2001): 23–44.

29 Tiffany Lee and Angela Kent, "Sexual addiction: Screening, assessment, diagnostic criteria, and treatment options," Western Michigan University, 2010.

30 Ibid.

31 David L. Delmonico, Donald Bubenzer, and John D. West, "Assessing sexual addiction with the sexual dependency inventory-revised," *Sexual Addiction & Compulsivity*, volume 5, issue 3 (1998): 179–86.

32 Patrick Carnes, Brad Green, and Stefanie Carnes, "The same yet different: Refocusing the sexual addiction screening test (SAST) to reflect orientation and gender," *Sexual Addiction & Compulsivity*, volume 17, issue 1 (2010): 7–30.

33 David W. Black, Laura L. D. Kehrberg, Denise L. Flumerfelt, and Steven S. Schlosser, "Characteristics of 36 subjects reporting compulsive sexual behavior," *American Journal of Psychiatry*, volume 154, issue 2 (1997): 243–250.

34 Tayla T. C. Lee, Kristine A. Ritchey, Jonathan D. Forbey, and George A. Gaither, "Psychometrics and comparison of the compulsive sexual behavior inventory and the sexual compulsivity scale in a male college student sample," *Sexual Addiction & Compulsivity*, volume 16, issue 2 (2009): 146–167.

35 Tiffany Lee and Angela Kent, "Sexual addiction: Screening, assessment, diagnostic criteria, & treatment options," Western Michigan University, 2010.

36 Ibid.

37 Richard Leedes, "The three most important criteria in diagnosing sexual addictions: Obsession, obsession, and obsession," *Sexual Addiction & Compulsivity*, volume 8 (2001): 216.

38 Michael Reece and Brian Dodge, "Exploring indicators of sexual compulsivity among men who cruise for sex on campus," *Sexual Addiction & Compulsivity*, volume 11 (2004): 87–113.

39 Richard Leedes, "The three most important criteria in diagnosing sexual addictions: Obsession, obsession, and obsession," *Sexual Addiction & Compulsivity*, volume 8 (2001): 215–26.

40 Tiffany Lee and Angela Kent, "Sexual addiction: Screening, assessment, diagnostic criteria, & treatment options," Western Michigan University, 2010.

41 Martin Plant and Moira Plant, "Sex addiction: A comparison with dependence on psychoactive drugs," *Journal of Substance Use*, volume 8, number 4 (2003): 260–266.

42 Matthew J. Del Giudice and Joshua Kutinsky, "Applying motivational interviewing to the treatment of sexual compulsivity and addiction," *Sexual Addiction & Compulsivity*, volume 14, issue 4 (2001): 303–19.

43 Tiffany Lee and Angela Kent, "Sexual addiction: Screening, assessment, diagnostic criteria, & treatment options," Western Michigan University, 2010.

44 Jan Parker and Diana Guest, "Individual sexual addiction treatment: A developmental perspective," *Sexual Addiction & Compulsivity*, volume 10, issue 1 (2003): 13–23.

45 Kenneth M. Adams and Donald W. Robinson, "Shame reduction, affect regulation, and sexual boundary development: Essential building blocks of sexual addiction treatment," *Sexual Addiction & Compulsivity*, volume 8, issue 1 (2001): 23–44.

46 Ibid.

BEHAVIORAL ADDICTION

47 Marie Wilson, "Creativity and shame reduction in sex addiction treatment," *Sexual Addiction & Compulsivity* 7 (2000): 229–48.

48 Lauren C. Spooner and William J. Lyddon, "Sandtray therapy for inpatient sexual addiction treatment: An application of constructivist change principles," *Journal of Constructivist Psychology* 20, no. 1 (2007): 53–85.

49 Marie Wilson, "Creativity and shame reduction in sex addiction treatment," *Sexual Addiction & Compulsivity* 7 (2000): 229–48.

50 Kenneth M. Adams and Donald W. Robinson, "Shame reduction, affect regulation, and sexual boundary development: Essential building blocks of sexual addiction treatment," *Sexual Addiction & Compulsivity* 8, no. 1 (2001): 23–44.

51 Jan Parker and Diana Guest, "Individual sexual addiction treatment: A developmental perspective," *Sexual Addiction & Compulsivity* 10, no. 1 (2003): 13–23.

52 Tiffany Lee and Angela Kent, "Sexual addiction: Screening, assessment, diagnostic criteria, & treatment options." Western Michigan University, 2010.

53 Martin Plant and Moira Plant, "Sex addiction: A comparison with dependence on psychoactive drugs," *Journal of Substance Use* 8, no. 4 (2003): 260–66.

CHAPTER FIVE

1 American Psychiatric Association, *Diagnostic and Statistical Manual of Mental Disorders, Fourth Edition, Text Revision* (Washington, DC: American Psychiatric Association, 2000).

2 Ruth H. Striegel-Moore and Debra L. Franko, "Should binge eating disorder be included in the DSM-V? A critical review of the state of the evidence," *Annual Review of Clinical Psychology* 4 (2008): 305–24.

3 Joshua I. Hrabosky, Robin M. Masheb, Marney A. White, and Carlos M. Grilo, "Overvaluation of shape and weight in binge eating disorder," *Journal of Consulting and Clinical Psychology* 75, no. 1 (2007): 175–80.

4 Nerissa L. Soh, Stephen W. Touyz, and Lois J. Surgenor, "Eating and body image disturbances across cultures: A review," *European Eating Disorders Review* 14, no. 1 (2006): 54–65.

5 Christopher G. Fairburn and Paul J. Harrison, "Eating disorders," *Lancet* 361, no. 9355 (2003): 407–16.

6 James I. Hudson, Eva Hiripi, Harrison G. Pope, Jr., and Ronald C. Kessler, "The prevalence and correlates of eating disorders in the National Comorbidity Survey Replication," *Biological Psychiatry* 61, no. 3 (2007): 348–58.

7 Robert L. Spitzer, Michael Devlin, B. Timothy Walsh, Deborah Hasin, Rena Wing, Marsha Marcus, Albert Stunkard, Thomas Wadden, Susan Yanovski, Stewart Agras, James Mitchell, and Cathy Nonas, "Binge eating disorder: A multisite field trial of the diagnostic criteria," *International Journal of Eating Disorders* 13, (1992): 191–203.

8 Ibid.

9 Substance Abuse and Mental Health Services Administration, Office of Applied Studies, "Results from the 2007 National Survey on Drug Use and Health: National Findings," (NSDUH Series H-34, DHHS Publication No. SMA 08-4343) (Rockville, MD: US Department of Health and Human Services) http://www.samhsa.gov/data/nsduh/ 2k7nsduh/2k7results.pdf (accessed June 11, 2012).

10 Barton J. Blinder, Edward J. Cumella, and Visant A. Sanathara, "Psychiatric

comorbidities of female inpatients with eating disorders," *Psychosomatic Medicine* 68 (2006): 454–62.

11 The National Center on Addiction and Substance Abuse (CASA) at Columbia University, "Food for thought: Substance abuse and eating disorders," (The National Center on Addiction and Substance Abuse (CASA) at Columbia University, 2003), http://www.casacolumbia.org/ templates/ Publications_Reports.aspx (accessed September 5, 2012).

12 Debra L. Franko, Pamela K. Keel, David J. Dorer, Mark A. Blais, Sherrie S. Delinsky, Kamryn T. Eddy, and David B. Herzog, "What predicts suicide attempts in women with eating disorders?," *Psychological Medicine* 34, no. 5 (2004): 843–53.

13 Sherry S. Stewart, Catrina G. Brown, Kristina Devoulyte, Jennifer Theakston, and Sarah E. Larsen, "Why do women with alcohol problems binge eat? Exploring connections between binge eating and heavy drinking in women receiving treatment for alcohol problems," *Journal of Health Psychology* 11, no. 3 (2006): 409–25.

14 Sarah P. Parkes, Elizabeth M. Saewyc, David N. Cox, and Laura J. MacKay, "Relationship between body image and stimulant use among Canadian adolescents," *Journal of Adolescent Health* 43, no. 6 (2008): 616–18.

15 David S. Goldbloom, Claudio A. Naranjo, Karen E. Bremner, and Lisa K. Hicks, "Eating disorders and alcohol abuse in women," *British Journal of Addiction* 87, no. 6 (1992): 913–19.

16 Joel D. Killen, C. Barr Taylor, Michael J. Telch, Thomas N. Robinson, David J. Maron, and Keith E. Saylor, "Depressive symptoms and substance use among adolescent binge eaters and purgers: A defined population study," *American Journal of Public Health*, volume 77, number 12 (1987): 1539–41.

17 Robert E. Frank, Mary K. Serdula, and Daniel Adame, "Weight loss and bulimic eating behavior: Changing patterns within a population of young adult women," *Southern Medical Journal* 84, no. 4 (1991): 457–60.

18 Cynthia M. Bulik, "Drug and alcohol abuse by bulimic women and their families," *American Journal of Psychiatry* 144, no. 12 (1987b): 1604–06.

19 Claire C. Holderness, Jeanne Brooks-Gunn, and Michelle P. Warren, "Co-morbidity of eating disorders and substance abuse: Review of the literature," *International Journal of Eating Disorders* 16, no. 1 (1994): 1–34.

20 James I. Hudson, Harrison G. Pope Jr., Jeffrey M. Jonas, and Deborah Yurgelun-Todd, "Family history study of anorexia nervosa and bulimia," *British Journal of Psychiatry* 142 (1983): 133–38.

21 Tammy L. Root, Andréa P. Pinheiro, Laura Thornton, Michael Strober, Fernando Fernandez-Aranda, Harry Brandt, Steve Crawford, Manfred M. Fichter, Katherine A. Halmi, Craig Johnson, Allan S. Kaplan, Kelly L. Klump, Maria La Via, James Mitchell, D. Blake Woodside, Alessandro Rotondo, Wade H. Berrettini, Walter H. Kaye, and Cynthia M. Bulik, "Substance use disorders in women with anorexia nervosa," *International Journal of Eating Disorders* 43, no. 1 (2010): 14–21.

22 Josefina Castro-Fornieles, Rosa Diaz, Javier Goti, Rosa Calvo, Laura Gonzalez, Lourdes Serrano, and Antoni Gual, "Prevalence and factors related to substance use among adolescents with eating disorders," *European Addiction Research* 16, no. 2 (2010): 61–68.

23 B. Timothy Walsh, Steven P. Roose, Alexander H. Glassman, Madeline Gladis, and Carla Sadik, "Bulimia and depression," *Psychosomatic Medicine* 47, no. 2 (1985): 123–31.

24 Michael Strober, Roberta Freeman, Stacy Bower, and Joanne Kigali, "Binge eating in anorexia nervosa predicts later onset of substance use disorder: A ten-year prospective, longitudinal follow-up of 95 adolescents," *Journal of Youth and Adolescence* 25, no. 4 (1996): 519–32.

25 David B. Herzog, Debra L. Franko, David J. Dorer, Pamela K. Keel, Safia Jackson, and Mary Pat Manzo, "Drug abuse in women with eating disorders," *International Journal of Eating Disorders* 39, no. 5 (2006): 364–68.

26 Lisa R. Cohen, Shelly F. Greenfield, Susan Gordon, Theresa Killeen, Huiping Jiang, Yulei Zhang, and Denise Hien, "Survey of eating disorder symptoms among women in treatment for substance abuse," *The American Journal on Addictions* 19, no. 3 (2010): 245–51.

27 F. Bonfà, S. Cabrini, M. Avanzi, O. Bettinardi, R. Spotti, and E. Uber, "Treatment dropout in drug-addicted women: Are eating disorders implicated?" *Eating and Weight Disorders* 13, no. 2 (2008): 81–86.

28 Robert Peveler and Christopher Fairburn, "Eating disorders in women who abuse alcohol," *British Journal of Addiction* 85, no. 12 (1990): 1633–38.

29 Claire C. Holderness, Jeanne Brooks-Gunn, and Michelle P. Warren, "Comorbidity of eating disorders and substance abuse: Review of the literature," *International Journal of Eating Disorders* 16, no. 1 (1994): 1–34.

30 M. D. Beary, J. H. Lacey, and Julius Merry, "Alcoholism and eating disorders in women of fertile age," *British Journal of Addiction* 81, no. 5 (1986): 685–89.

31 Sarah P. Parkes, Elizabeth M. Saewyc, David N. Cox, and Laura J. MacKay, "Relationship between body image and stimulant use among Canadian adolescents," *Journal of Adolescent Health* 43, no. 6 (2008): 616–18.

32 Ellen R. Gritz and Lori A. Crane, "Use of diet pills and amphetamines to lose weight among smoking and nonsmoking high school seniors," *Health Psychology* 10, no. 5 (1991): 330–35.

33 Mary-Lynn Brecht, Ann O'Brien, Christina von Mayrhauser, and M. Douglas Anglin, "Methamphetamine use behaviors and gender differences," *Addictive Behaviors* 29, no. 1 (2004): 89–106.

34 Susan G. Sherman, Danielle German, Bangorn Sirirojn, Nick Thompson, Apinun Aramrattana, and David D. Celentano, "Initiation of methamphetamine use among young Thai drug users: A qualitative study," *Journal of Adolescent Health* 42, no. 1 (2008): 36–42.

35 Sarah L. Welch and Christopher G. Fairburn, "Impulsivity or comorbidity in bulimia nervosa: A controlled study of deliberate self-harm and alcohol and drug misuse in a community sample," *British Journal of Psychiatry* 169, no. 4 (1996): 451–58.

36 Carlos M. Grilo, Marney A. White, and Robin M. Masheb, "DSM-IV psychiatric disorder comorbidity and its correlates in binge eating disorder," *International Journal of Eating Disorders* 42, no. 3 (2009): 228–34.

37 Gloria M. Miele, Sarah M. Tilly, Michael First, and Allen Frances, "The definition of dependence and behavioral addictions," *British Journal of Addiction* 85 (1990): 1421–23.

38 Aviel Goodman, "Addiction: Definition and implications," *British Journal of Addiction* 85 (1990): 1403–08.

39 G. Terence Wilson, "Eating disorders and addiction," *Drugs & Society* 15, no. 1 (2000): 87–101.

40 Stephanie E. Cassin and Kristin M. von Ranson, "Is binge eating experienced as an addiction?" *Appetite* 49, no. 3 (2007): 687–90.

41 Ruth H. Striegel-Moore, Lisa R. Silberstein, and Judith Rodin, "The social self in bulimia nervosa: Public self-consciousness, social anxiety, and perceived fraudulence," *Journal of Abnormal Psychology* 102, no. 2 (1993): 297–303.

42 George F. Koob, and Michel Le Moal, "Drug addiction, dysregulation of reward, and allostasis," *Neuropsychopharmacology* 24, no. 2 (2001): 97–129.

43 V. M. Lingswiler, J. H. Crowther, and M. A. Stephens, "Affective and cognitive antecedents to eating episodes in bulimia and binge eating," *International Journal of Eating Disorders* 8, no. 5 (1989): 533–39.

44 Jessica H. Baker, Suzanne E. Mazzeo, and Kenneth S. Kendler, "Association between broadly defined bulimia nervosa and drug use disorders: Common genetic and environmental influences," *International Journal of Eating Disorders* 40, no. 8 (2007): 673–78.

45 Constance Holden, "'Behavioral' addictions: Do they exist?" *Science* 249, no. 5544 (2001): 980–82.

46 G. Terence Wilson, "Eating disorders, obesity and addiction," *European Eating Disorders Review* 18, no. 5 (2010): 341–51.

47 Sharon Dawe and Natalie J. Loxton, "The role of impulsivity in the development of substance use and eating disorders," *Neuroscience and Biobehavioral Reviews* 28, no. 3 (2004): 343–51.

48 Wendy L. Wolfe, and Stephen A. Maisto, "The relationship between eating disorders and substance use: Moving beyond co-prevalence research," *Clinical Psychology Review* 20, no. 5 (2000): 617–31.

49 Kathleen R. Merikangas, Marilyn Stolar, Denise E. Stevens, Joseph Goulet, Martin A. Preisig, Brenda Fenton, Heping Zhang, Stephanie S. O'Malley, and Bruce J. Rounsaville, "Familial transmission of substance use disorders," *Archives of General Psychiatry* 55 (1998): 973–79.

50 Ibid.

51 Graham W. Redgrave, Janelle W. Coughlin, Leslie J. Heinberg, and Angela S. Guarda, "First-degree relative history of alcoholism in eating disorder inpatients: Relationship to eating and substance use pathology," *Eating Behaviors* 8, no. 1 (2007): 15–22.

52 Robert L. Spitzer, Michael Devlin, B. Timothy Walsh, Deborah Hasin, Rena Wing, Marsha Marcus, Albert Stunkard, Thomas Wadden, Susan Yanovski, Stewart Agras, James Mitchell, and Cathy Nonas, "Binge eating disorder: A multisite field trial of the diagnostic criteria," *International Journal of Eating Disorders* 13, (1992): 191–203.

53 Glenn Waller and Rachel Calam, "Parenting and family factors in eating problems," in *Understanding Eating Disorders: Anorexia Nervosa, Bulimia Nervosa, and Obesity*, ed. by LeeAnn Alexander-Mott and D. Barry Lumsden (Washington, DC: Taylor & Francis, 1994), 61–76.

54 Salvador Minuchin, Bernice L. Rosman, and Lester Baker, *Psychosomatic Families: Anorexia Nervosa in Context* (Cambridge, MA: Harvard University Press, 1978).

55 Renee R. Hoste and Daniel le Grange, "Expressed emotion among white and ethnic minority families of adolescents with bulimia nervosa," *European Eating Disorders Review* 16, no. 5 (2008): 395–400.

56 K. M. Pike, A. Hilbert, Denise E. Wilfley, C. G. Fairburn, F. A. Dohm, B. T. Walsh, and R. H. Striegel-Moore, "Toward an understanding of risk factors for anorexia nervosa: A case-controlled study," *Psychological Medicine* 38, no. 10 (2008): 1443–53.

57 Claire V. Wiseman, Suzanne R. Sunday, Patricia Halligan, Suzanne Korn, Christine Brown, and Katherine A. Halmi, "Substance dependence and eating disorders: Impact of sequence on comorbidity," *Comprehensive Psychiatry* 40, no. 5 (1999): 332–36.

58 Nora D. Volkow, Gene-Jack Wang, and Ruben D. Baler, "Reward, dopamine and the control of food intake: Implications for obesity," *Trends in Cognitive Sciences* 15, no. 1 (2011): 37–46.

59 Dean D. Krahn, "The relationship between eating disorders and substance abuse," *Journal of Substance Abuse* 3, no. 2 (1991): 239–53.

60 Ibid.

61 M. E. Carroll, C. P. France, and R. A. Meisch, "Food deprivation increases oral and intravenous drug intake in rats," *Science* 205, no. 4403 (1979): 319–21.

62 Cynthia M. Bulik and Emma C. Brinded, "The effect of food deprivation on alcohol consumption in bulimic and control women," *Addiction* 88, no. 11 (1993): 1545–51.

63 Sherry H. Stewart, Maria Angelopoulos, Jan M. Baker, and Fred J. Boland, "Relations between dietary restraint and patterns of alcohol use in young adult women," *Psychology of Addictive Behaviors*, volume 14, issue 1 (2000): 77–82.

64 Darla E. Kendzor, Lauren E. Baillie, Claire E. Adams, Diana W. Stewart, and Amy L. Copeland, "The effect of food deprivation on cigarette smoking in females," *Addictive Behavior* 33, no. 10 (2008): 1353–59.

65 M. D. Beary, J. H. Lacey, and Julius Merry, "Alcoholism and eating disorders in women of fertile age," *British Journal of Addiction* 81, no. 5 (1986): 685–89.

66 Asli Çepik, Zehra Arikan, Cumhar Boratav, and Erdal Lsik, "Bulimia in a male alcoholic: A symptom substitution in alcoholism," *International Journal of Eating Disorders* 17, no. 2 (1995): 201–04.

67 Claire C. Holderness, Jeanne Brooks-Gunn, and Michelle P. Warren, "Co-morbidity of eating disorders and substance abuse: Review of the literature," *International Journal of Eating Disorders* 16, no. 1 (1994): 1–34.

68 H. Valerie Curran and Katy Robjant, "Eating attitudes, weight concerns, and beliefs about drug effects in women who use ecstasy," *Journal of Psychopharmacology* 20, no. 3 (2006): 425–31.

69 Eric J. Button, Bhanu Chadalavada, and Robert L. Palmer, "Mortality and predictors of death in a cohort of patients presenting to an eating disorder service," *International Journal of Eating Disorders*, volume 43, issue 5 (2010): 387–92.

70 Ibid.

71 A. H. Conason, A. Brunstein Klomek, and L. Sher, "Recognizing alcohol and drug abuse in patients with eating disorders," *Quarterly Journal of Medicine* 99 (2006): 335–39.

72 Melanie A. Katzman, Art Greenberg, and Ivy D. Marcus, "Bulimia in opiate-addicted women: Developmental cousin and relapse factor," *Journal of Substance Abuse Treatment* 8, no. 3 (1991): 107–12.

73 Debra L. Franko, David J. Dorer, Pamela K. Keel, Safia Jackson, Mary Pat Manzo, and David B. Herzog, "How do eating disorders and alcohol use disorder influence each other?," *International Journal of Eating Disorders* 38, no. 3 (2000): 200–07.

74 Cynthia L. Alexander, "Transfer of Addiction (Transfer of Vice), Alcohol, and Smoking," in *The Emotional First + Aid Kit. A Practical Guide to Life After Bariatric Surgery* (Second Ed.) (West Chester, PA, Matrix Medical Communications, 2009: 136).

75 Margaret H. Emerson, Ellen Glovsky, Hortensia Amaro, and Rita Nieves, "Unhealthy weight gain during treatment for alcohol and drug use in four residential programs for Latina and African American women," *Substance Use and Misuse* 4, no. 11 (2009): 1553–65.

76 Robert W. Jeffery, Deborah J. Hennrikus, Harry A. Lando, David M. Murray, and Jane W. Liu, "Reconciling conflicting findings regarding postcessation weight concerns and success in smoking cessation," *Health Psychology* 19, no. 3 (2000): 242–46.

77 Food and Drug Administration. *Desoxyn: Methamphetamine Hydrochloride Tablets, USP*. Med Guide (2007). Retrieved from http://www.accessdata.fda.gov/ drugsatfda_docs/label/2007/ 005378s026lbl.pdf

78 Suzette Glasner-Edwards, Larissa J. Mooney, Patricia Marinelli-Casey, Maureen Hillhouse, Alfonso Ang, Richard Rawson, and The Methamphetamine Treatment Project Corporate Authors, "Bulimia nervosa among methamphetamine dependent adults: Association with outcomes three years after treatment," *Eating Disorders* 19, no. 3 (2011): 259–69.

79 Susan G. Sherman, Danielle German, Bangorn Sirirojn, Nick Thompson, Apinun Aramrattana, and David D. Celentano, "Initiation of methamphetamine use among young Thai drug users: A qualitative study," *Journal of Adolescent Health* 42, no. 1 (2008): 36–42.

80 Rachel Gonzales, Larissa Mooney, and Richard A. Rawson, "The methamphetamine problem in the United States," *Annual Review of Public Health* 31 (2010): 385–98.

81 Janine L. Pillitteri, Saul Shiffman, Jeffrey M. Rohay, Andrea M. Harkins, Steven L. Burton, and Thomas A. Wadden, "Use of dietary supplements for weight loss in the United States: Results of a national survey," *Obesity* 16, no. 4 (2008): 790–96.

82 Carlos M. Grilo, Rajita Sinha, and Stephanie S. O'Malley, "Eating disorders and alcohol use disorders," *Alcohol Health and Research World* 26, no. 2 (2002): 151–60.

83 Susan Merle Gordon, J. Aaron Johnson, Shelly F. Greenfield, Lisa Cohen, Therese Killeen, and Paul M. Roman, "Assessment and treatment of co-occurring eating disorders in publicly funded addiction treatment programs," *Psychiatric Services* 59, no. 9 (2008): 1056–59.

84 Anne R. Lindsay, Courtney S. Warren, Sara C. Velasquez, and Minggen Lu, "A gender-specific approach to improving substance abuse treatment for women: The Healthy Steps to Freedom (HSF) program," *Journal of Substance Abuse Treatment,* 43, (2012): 61–69.

85 Robyn Sysko and Tom Hildebrandt, "Cognitive-behavioural therapy for individuals with bulimia nervosa and a co-occurring substance use disorder," *European Eating Disorders Review* 17, no. 2 (2009): 89–100.

CHAPTER SIX

1 Benjamin J. Sadock and Virginia A. Sadock, "Impulse-Control Disorders Not Elsewhere Classified," in *Kaplan & Sadock's Synopsis of Psychiatry: Behavioral Sciences/Clinical Psychiatry, Tenth Edition* (Philadelphia, PA: Lippincott Williams & Wilkins, 2007), 773–85.

2 American Psychiatric Association, *Diagnostic and Statistical Manual of Mental Disorders, Fourth Edition, Text Revision* (Washington, DC: American Psychiatric Association, 2000).

3 Benjamin J. Sadock and Virginia A. Sadock, "Impulse-Control Disorders Not Elsewhere Classified," in *Kaplan & Sadock's Synopsis of Psychiatry: Behavioral Sciences/Clinical Psychiatry, Tenth Edition* (Philadelphia, PA: Lippincott Williams & Wilkins, 2007), 773–85.

4 Eric Hollander, Heather Berlin, and Dan Stein, "Impulse-Control Disorders Not Elsewhere Classified," in *The American Psychiatric Publishing Textbook of Psychiatry, Fifth Edition*, by Marc Galanter and Herbert D. Kleber (Washington, DC: American Psychiatric Publishing, Inc., 2008).

5 Jon E. Grant, Kyle A. Williams, and Marc N. Potenza, "Impulse control disorders in adolescent psychiatric inpatients: Co-occurring disorders and sex differences," *Journal of Clinical Psychiatry* 68 (2007): 1584–92.

6 Eric Hollander, Heather Berlin, and Dan Stein, "Impulse-Control Disorders Not Elsewhere Classified," in *The American Psychiatric Publishing Textbook of Psychiatry, Fifth Edition*, by Marc Galanter and Herbert D. Kleber (Washington, DC: American Psychiatric Publishing, Inc., 2008).

7 Benjamin J. Sadock and Virginia A. Sadock, "Impulse-Control Disorders Not Elsewhere Classified," in *Kaplan & Sadock's Synopsis of Psychiatry: Behavioral Sciences/Clinical Psychiatry, Tenth Edition* (Philadelphia, PA: Lippincott Williams & Wilkins, 2007), 773–85.

8 Eric Hollander, Heather Berlin, Dan Stein, "Impulse-Control Disorders Not Elsewhere Classified," in *The American Psychiatric Publishing Textbook of Psychiatry, Fifth Edition*, by Marc Galanter and Herbert D. Kleber (Washington, DC: American Psychiatric Publishing, Inc., 2008).

9 Ibid.

10 W. Gordon Frankle, Ilise Lombardo, Antonia S. New, Marianne Goodman, Peter S. Talbot, Yiyun Huang, Dah-Ren Hwang, Mark Slifstein, Susan Curry, Anissa Abi-Dargham, Marc Laruelle, and Larry J. Siever, "Brain serotonin transporter distribution in subjects with impulsive Aggressivity: A positron emission study with [^{11}C] McN 5652," *American Journal of Psychiatry* 162, no. 5 (2005): 915–23.

11 Larry J. Siever, "Neurobiology of aggression and violence," *American Journal of Psychiatry* 165, no. 4 (2008): 429–42.

12 Eric Hollander, Heather Berlin, Dan Stein, "Impulse-Control Disorders Not Elsewhere Classified," in *The American Psychiatric Publishing Textbook of Psychiatry, Fifth Edition*, by Marc Galanter and Herbert D. Kleber (Washington, DC: American Psychiatric Publishing, Inc., 2008).

13 Emil F. Coccaro, Royce J. Lee, and Richard J. Kavoussi, "A double-blind, randomized, placebo-controlled trial of fluoxetine in patients with intermittent Explosive Disorder," *Journal of Clinical Psychiatry* 70, no. 5 (2009): 653–62.

14 Bernardo Dell'Osso, A. Carlo Altamura, Andrea Allen, Donatella Marazziti, and Eric Hollander, "Epidemiologic and clinical updates on impulse control disorders: A critical review," *European Archives of Psychiatry Clinical Neuroscience* 256 (2006): 464–75.

15 Larry J. Siever, "Neurobiology of aggression and violence," *American Journal of Psychiatry* 165, no. 4 (2008): 429–42.

16 Michael S. McCloskey, Kurtis L. Noblett, Jerry L. Deffenbacher, Jackie K. Gollan, and Emil F. Coccaro, "Cognitive-behavioral therapy for intermittent explosive disorder: A pilot randomized clinical trial," *Journal of Consulting and Clinical Psychology* 76, no. 5 (2008): 876–86.

17 American Psychiatric Association, *Diagnostic and Statistical Manual of Mental Disorders, Fourth Edition, Text Revision* (Washington, DC: American Psychiatric Association, 2000).

18 Benjamin J. Sadock and Virginia A. Sadock, "Impulse-Control Disorders Not Elsewhere Classified," in *Kaplan & Sadock's Synopsis of Psychiatry: Behavioral Sciences/Clinical Psychiatry, Tenth Edition* (Philadelphia, PA: Lippincott Williams & Wilkins, 2007), 773–85.

19 Carlos Blanco, Jon Grant, Nancy M. Petry, H. Blair Simpson, Analucia A. Alegria, Shang-Min Liu, and Deborah Hasin, "Prevalence and correlates of shoplifting in the United States: Results from the National Epidemiological Survey on Alcohol and Related Conditions (NESARC)," *American Journal of Psychiatry* 165, no. 7 (2008): 905–13.

20 Jon E. Grant, Kyle A. Williams, and Marc N. Potenza, "Impulse control disorders in adolescent psychiatric inpatients: Co-occurring disorders and sex differences," *Journal of Clinical Psychiatry*, volume 68 (2007): 1584–92.

21 Jon E. Grant, Laura Levine, Daniel Kim, and Marc N. Potenza, "Impulse control disorders in adult psychiatric inpatients," *American Journal of Psychiatry* 162, no. 11 (2005): 2184–88.

22 Brian L. Odlaug and Jon E. Grant, "Impulse-control disorders in a college sample: Results from the self-administered Minnesota Impulse Disorders Interview (MIDI)," *Primary Care Companion Journal of Clinical Psychiatry* 12, no. 2 (2010): e1–e5.

23 Eric Hollander, Heather Berlin, Dan Stein, "Impulse-Control Disorders Not Elsewhere Classified, in *The American Psychiatric Publishing Textbook of*

Psychiatry, Fifth Edition, by Marc Galanter and Herbert D. Kleber (Washington, DC: American Psychiatric Publishing, Inc., 2008).

24 Jon E. Grant and Marc N. Potenza, "Gender-related differences in individuals seeking treatment for kleptomania," *CNS Spectrum* 13, no. 3 (2008): 235–45.

25 Eric Hollander, Heather Berlin, Dan Stein, "Impulse-Control Disorders Not Elsewhere Classified," in *The American Psychiatric Publishing Textbook of Psychiatry, Fifth Edition,* by Marc Galanter and Herbert D. Kleber (Washington, DC: American Psychiatric Publishing, Inc., 2008).

26 Franck J. Baylé, Hervé Caci, Bruno Millet, Sami Richa, and Jean-Pierre Olié, "Psychopathology and comorbidity of psychiatric disorders in patients with kleptomania," *American Journal of Psychiatry* 160, no. 8 (2003): 1509–13.

27 Jon E. Grant and Marc N. Potenza, "Gender-related differences in individuals seeking treatment for kleptomania," *CNS Spectrum* 13, no. 3 (2008): 235–45.

28 Benjamin J. Sadock and Virginia A. Sadock, "Impulse-Control Disorders Not Elsewhere Classified," in *Kaplan & Sadock's Synopsis of Psychiatry: Behavioral Sciences/Clinical Psychiatry, Tenth Edition* (Philadelphia, PA: Lippincott Williams & Wilkins, 2007), 773–85.

29 Jon E. Grant, Brian L. Odlaug, and Jeffrey R. Wozniak, "Neuropsychological functioning in kleptomania," *Behavior Research and Therapy* 45, no. 7 (2007): 1663–70.

30 Jon E. Grant, Stephen Correia, and Thea Brennan-Krohn, "White matter integrity in kleptomania: A pilot study," *Psychiatry Research: Neuroimaging* 147, nos. 2-3 (2006): 233–37.

31 Benjamin J. Sadock and Virginia A. Sadock, "Impulse-Control Disorders Not Elsewhere Classified," in *Kaplan & Sadock's Synopsis of Psychiatry: Behavioral Sciences/Clinical Psychiatry, Tenth Edition* (Philadelphia, PA: Lippincott Williams & Wilkins, 2007), 773–85.

32 Eric Hollander, Heather Berlin, and Dan Stein, "Impulse-Control Disorders Not Elsewhere Classified," in *The American Psychiatric Publishing Textbook of Psychiatry, Fifth Edition,* by Marc Galanter and Herbert D. Kleber (Washington, DC: American Psychiatric Publishing, Inc., 2008).

33 Benjamin J. Sadock and Virginia A. Sadock, "Impulse-Control Disorders Not Elsewhere Classified," in *Kaplan & Sadock's Synopsis of Psychiatry: Behavioral Sciences/Clinical Psychiatry, Tenth Edition* (Philadelphia, PA: Lippincott Williams & Wilkins, 2007), 773–85.

34 Eric Hollander, Heather Berlin, and Dan Stein, "Impulse-Control Disorders Not Elsewhere Classified," in *The American Psychiatric Publishing Textbook of Psychiatry, Fifth Edition,* by Marc Galanter and Herbert D. Kleber (Washington, DC: American Psychiatric Publishing, Inc., 2008).

35 Lorrin M. Koran, Dana Bodnik, and Pinhas N. Dannon, "Kleptomania: Clinical Aspects," in *Impulse Control Disorders,* ed. by Elias Aboujaoude and Lorrin Koran (New York: Cambridge University Press, 2010), 34–50.

36 James E. Mitchell, Melissa Burgard, Ron Faber, Ross D. Crosby, and Martina de Zwaan, "Cognitive behavioral therapy for compulsive buying disorder," *Behaviour Research and Therapy* 44, no. 12 (2006): 1859–65.

37 Lorrin M. Koran, Dana Bodnik, and Pinhas N. Dannon, "Kleptomania: Clinical Aspects," *Impulse Control Disorders,* ed. by Elias Aboujaoude and Lorrin Koran (New York: Cambridge University Press, 2010), 34–50.

38 Liana Schreiber, Brian L. Odlaug, and Jon E. Grant, "Impulse control disorders: Updated review of clinical characteristics and pharmacological management," *Frontiers in Psychiatry* 2, art. no. 1 (2011): 1–11.

39 Jon E. Grant, Suck Won Kim and Brian Odlaug, "A double-blind, placebo-

controlled study of the opiate antagonist, naltrexone, in the treatment of kleptomania," *Biological Psychiatry* 65, no. 7 (2009): 600–06.

40 Farid Ramzi Talih, "Kleptomania and potential exacerbating factors: A review and case report," *Innovations in Clinical Neuroscience* 8, no. 10 (2011): 35–39.

41 American Psychiatric Association, *Diagnostic and Statistical Manual of Mental Disorders, Fourth Edition, Text Revision* (Washington, DC: American Psychiatric Association, 2000).

42 Eric Hollander, Heather Berlin, and Dan Stein, "Impulse-Control Disorders Not Elsewhere Classified," in *The American Psychiatric Publishing Textbook of Psychiatry, Fifth Edition*, by Marc Galanter and Herbert D. Kleber (Washington, DC: American Psychiatric Publishing, Inc., 2008).

43 Benjamin J. Sadock and Virginia A. Sadock, "Impulse-Control Disorders Not Elsewhere Classified," in *Kaplan & Sadock's Synopsis of Psychiatry: Behavioral Sciences/Clinical Psychiatry, Tenth Edition* (Philadelphia, PA: Lippincott Williams & Wilkins, 2007), 773–85.

44 Eric Hollander, Heather Berlin, and Dan Stein, "Impulse-Control Disorders Not Elsewhere Classified," in *The American Psychiatric Publishing Textbook of Psychiatry, Fifth Edition*, by Marc Galanter and Herbert D. Kleber (Washington, DC: American Psychiatric Publishing, Inc., 2008).

45 Bernardo Dell'Osso, A. Carlo Altamura, Andrea Allen, Donatella Marazziti, and Eric Hollander, "Epidemiologic and clinical updates on impulse control disorders: A critical review," *European Archives of Psychiatry Clinical Neuroscience* 256 (2006): 464–75.

46 Carlos Blanco, Analucia A. Alegria, Nancy M. Petry, Jon E. Grant, H. Blair Simpson, Shang-Min Liu, Bridget F. Grant, and Deborah S. Hasin, "Prevalence and correlates of fire-setting in the United States: Results from the National Epidemiological Survey on Alcohol and Related Conditions (NESARC)," *Journal of Clinical Psychiatry* 71, no. 9 (2010): 1218–25.

47 Brian L. Odlaug and Jon E. Grant, "Impulse-control disorders in a college sample: Results from the self-administered Minnesota Impulse Disorders Interview (MIDI)," *Primary Care Companion Journal of Clinical Psychiatry* 12, no. 2 (2010): e1–e5.

48 Jon E. Grant, Laura Levine, Daniel Kim, and Marc N. Potenza, "Impulse control disorders in adult psychiatric inpatients," *American Journal of Psychiatry* 162, no. 11 (2005): 2184–88.

49 Jon E. Grant, Kyle A. Williams, and Marc N. Potenza, "Impulse control disorders in adolescent psychiatric inpatients: Co-occurring disorders and sex differences," *Journal of Clinical Psychiatry* 68 (2007): 1584–92.

50 Benjamin J. Sadock and Virginia A. Sadock, "Impulse-Control Disorders Not Elsewhere Classified," in *Kaplan & Sadock's Synopsis of Psychiatry: Behavioral Sciences/Clinical Psychiatry, Tenth Edition* (Philadelphia, PA: Lippincott Williams & Wilkins 2007), 773–85.

51 Jon E. Grant and Suck Won Kim, "Clinical characteristics and psychiatric comorbidity of pyromania," *Journal of Clinical Psychiatry* 68 (2007): 1717–22.

52 Matti Virkkunen, Monika Eggert, Robert Rawlings, and Markku Linnoila, "A prospective follow-up study of alcoholic violent offenders and fire setters," *Archives of General Psychiatry* 53 (1996): 523–29.

53 Jon E. Grant, "SPECT imaging and treatment of pyromania," *Journal of Clinical Psychiatry* 67, no. 6 (2006): 998.

54 Eric Hollander, Heather Berlin, Dan Stein, "Impulse-Control Disorders Not Elsewhere Classified," *The American Psychiatric Publishing Textbook of Psychiatry, Fifth Edition*, by Marc Galanter and Herbert D. Kleber (Washington, DC: American Psychiatric Publishing, Inc., 2008).

55 Bernardo Dell'Osso, A. Carlo Altamura, Andrea Allen, Donatella Marazziti, and Eric Hollander, "Epidemiologic and clinical updates on impulse control disorders: A critical review," *European Archives of Psychiatry Clinical Neuroscience* 256 (2006): 464–75.

56 Jon E. Grant, "SPECT imaging and treatment of pyromania," *Journal of Clinical Psychiatry* 67, no. 6 (2006): 998.

57 Jon E. Grant and Suck Won Kim, "Clinical characteristics and psychiatric comorbidity of pyromania," *Journal of Clinical Psychiatry* 68 (2007): 1717–22.

58 Eric Hollander, Heather Berlin, and Dan Stein, "Impulse-Control Disorders Not Elsewhere Classified," in *The American Psychiatric Publishing Textbook of Psychiatry, Fifth Edition*, by Marc Galanter and Herbert D. Kleber (Washington, DC: American Psychiatric Publishing, Inc., 2008).

59 Samuel R. Chamberlain, Lara Menzies, Barbara J. Sahakian, and Naomi A. Fineberg, "Lifting the veil on trichotillomania," *American Journal of Psychiatry* 164, no. 4, (2007): 568–74.

60 Jon E. Grant and Brian L. Odlaug, "Clinical characteristics of trichotillomania with trichophagia," *Comprehensive Psychiatry* 49, no. 6 (2008): 579–84.

61 Benjamin J. Sadock and Virginia A. Sadock, "Impulse-Control Disorders Not Elsewhere Classified," in *Kaplan & Sadock's Synopsis of Psychiatry: Behavioral Sciences/Clinical Psychiatry, Tenth Edition* (Philadelphia, PA: Lippincott Williams & Wilkins, 2007), 773–85.

62 Samuel R. Chamberlain, Lara Menzies, Barbara J. Sahakian, and Naomi A. Fineberg, "Lifting the veil on trichotillomania," *American Journal of Psychiatry* 164, no. 4, (2007): 568–74.

63 Ibid.

64 Ibid.

65 Samuel R. Chamberlain, Brian L. Odlaug, Vasileios Boulougouris, Naomi Fineberg, and Jon E. Grant, "Trichotillomania: Neurobiology and treatment," *Neuroscience and Biobehavioral Reviews* 33 (2009): 831–42.

66 Ibid.

67 Samuel R. Chamberlain, Lara Menzies, Barbara J. Sahakian, and Naomi A. Fineberg, "Lifting the veil on trichotillomania," *American Journal of Psychiatry* 164, no. 4, (2007): 568–74.

68 Kathleen Trainor, "Treating trichotillomania in children and adolescents: CBT versus medication," *American Journal of Psychiatry* 164, no. 10 (2007): 1610–11.

69 Samuel R. Chamberlain, Brian L. Odlaug, Vasileios Boulougouris, Naomi Fineberg, and Jon E. Grant, "Trichotillomania: Neurobiology and treatment," *Neuroscience and Biobehavioral Reviews* 33 (2009): 831–42.

70 Ibid.

71 Jon E. Grant, Brian L. Odlaug, and Suck Won Kim, "N-Acetylcysteine, a glutamate modulator, in the treatment of trichotillomania," *Archives of General Psychiatry* 66, no. 7 (2009): 756–63.

72 Michael R. Walther, Benjamin T. P. Tucker, and Douglas W. Woods, "Trichotillomania: Clinical Aspects," in *Impulse Control Disorders*, ed. by Elias Aboujaoude and Lorrin M. Koran (New York: Cambridge University Press, 2010), 97–110.

73 Benjamin J. Sadock and Virginia A. Sadock, "Impulse-Control Disorders Not Elsewhere Classified," in *Kaplan & Sadock's Synopsis of Psychiatry: Behavioral Sciences/Clinical Psychiatry, Tenth Edition* (Philadelphia, PA: Lippincott Williams & Wilkins, 2007), 773–85.

74 Eric Hollander, Heather Berlin, and Dan Stein, "Impulse-Control Disorders

Not Elsewhere Classified," in *The American Psychiatric Publishing Textbook of Psychiatry, Fifth Edition*, by Marc Galanter and Herbert D. Kleber (Washington, DC: American Psychiatric Publishing, Inc., 2008).

75 Benjamin J. Sadock and Virginia A. Sadock, "Impulse-Control Disorders Not Elsewhere Classified," in *Kaplan & Sadock's Synopsis of Psychiatry: Behavioral Sciences/Clinical Psychiatry, Tenth Edition* (Philadelphia, PA: Lippincott Williams & Wilkins, 2007), 773–85.

76 Jon E. Grant, "The Relationship of Impulse Control Disorders to Drug and Alcohol Addiction," in *Impulse Control Disorders: A Clinician's Guide to Understanding and Treating Behavioral Addictions*, by Jon E. Grant (New York: W. W. Norton & Company, 2008), 45–58.

77 Jon E. Grant, Suck Won Kim and Brian Odlaug, "A double-blind, placebo-controlled study of the opiate antagonist, naltrexone, in the treatment of kleptomania," *Biological Psychiatry* 65, no. 7 (2009): 600–06.

78 Eric Hollander, Bryann Baker, Jessica Kahn, and Dan Stein, "Conceptualizing and Assessing Impulse-Control Disorders," in *Clinical Manual of Impulse-Control Disorders*, ed. by Eric Hollander and Dan Stein (Washington DC: American Psychiatric Publishing, Inc., 2006), 1–18.

79 http://www.dsm5.org/ProposedRevision, accessed March 31, 2012.

CHAPTER SEVEN

1 Ronald Pies, "Should DSM-V designate "Internet addiction" a mental disorder?," *Psychiatry* 6, no. 2 (2009): 31–37.

2 Nancy, M. Petry, "Commentary on Van Rooij et al. (2011): 'Gaming addiction'—a psychiatric disorder or not?" *Addiction* 106, no. 1 (2011): 213.

3 Karin H. Bergmark, Anders Bergmark, and Olle Findahl, "Extensive Internet involvement—Addiction or emerging lifestyle?," *International Journal of Environmental Research and Public Health* 8 (2011): 4488–4501.

4 Rita Rubin, "Psychologists Challenge Proposed New Diagnosis in DSM-5," *USA Today*, November 10, 2011. http://yourlife.usatoday.com/health/medical/metnalhealth/ story/2011-11-09/Psychologiest-challenge-proposed-new-diagnoses-in-DSM-5/51144104/1 (accessed April 4, 2012).

5 Ronald Pies, "Should DSM-V designate "Internet addiction" a mental disorder?" *Psychiatry* 6, no. 2 (2009): 31–37.

6 Martha Shaw and Donald W. Black, "Internet addiction: Definition, assessment, epidemiology and clinical management," *CNS Drugs* 22, no. 5 (2008): 353–65.

7 Elias Aboujaoude, Foreword, in *Internet Addiction: A Handbook and Guide to Evaluation and Treatment*, ed. by Kimberly S. Young and Christiano Nabuco de Abreu (Hoboken, NJ: John Wiley & Sons, Inc., 2011), viii.

8 Nathan A. Shapira, Mary C. Lessig, Toby D. Goldsmith, Steven T. Szabo, Martin Lazoritz, Mark S. Gold, and Dan J. Stein, "Problematic internet use: Proposed classification and diagnostic criteria," *Depression and Anxiety* 17, no. 4 (2003): 214.

9 Ronald Pies, "Should DSM-V designate "Internet addiction" a mental disorder?" *Psychiatry* 6, no. 2 (2009): 31–37.

10 Martha Shaw and Donald W. Black, "Internet addiction: Definition, assessment, epidemiology and clinical management," *CNS Drugs* 22, no. 5 (2008): 355.

11 Kimberly S. Young and Christiano Nabuco de Abreu, eds., *Internet Addiction: A Handbook and Guide to Evaluation and Treatment* (Hoboken, NJ: John Wiley & Sons, Inc., 2011).

12 Kimberly S. Young, "Assessment and treatment of problem Internet use," in *The Oxforedc Handbook of Impulse Control Disorders,* ed. Jon E. Grant and Mark N. Potenza (New York: Oxford University Press, 2012), 389–97.

13 Janet Morahan-Martin and Phyllis Schumacher, "Incidence and correlates of pathological internet use among college students," *Computers in Human Behavior* 16, no. 1 (2000): 13–29.

14 Elias Aboujaoude, Lorrin M. Koran, Nona Gamel, Michael D. Large, and Richard T. Serpe, "Potential markers for problematic internet use: a telephone survey of 2,513 adults," *CNS Spectrums* 11, no. 10 (2006): 750–55.

15 Ibid. 752

16 Inger J. Bakken, Hanne, G. Wenzel, K. Gunnar Gotestam, Agneta Johansson, and Anita Oren, "Internet addiction among Norwegian adults: A stratified probability sample study," *Scandinavian Journal of Psychology* 50 (2009): 121–27.

17 Janet Morahan-Martin and Phyllis Schumacher, "Incidence and correlates of pathological Internet use among college students," *Computers in Human Behavior* 16, no. 1 (2000): 13–29.

18 Douglas Gentile, "Pathological video-game use among youth ages 8 to 18," *Psychological Science* 20, no. 5 (2009): 594–602.

19 Lawrence T. Lam, Zi-wen Peng, Jin-cheng Mai, Jin Jing, "Factors associated with Internet addiction among adolescents," *CyberPsychology & Behavior* 12, no. 5 (2009): 551–55.

20 Nazir S. Hawi, "Internet addiction among adolescents in Lebanon," *Computers in Human Behavior* 28, no. 3 (2012): 1046.

21 Soo Kyung Park, Jae Yop Kim, and Choon Bum Cho, "Prevalence of Internet addiction and correlations with family factors among South Korean adolescents," *Adolescence* 43, no. 172 (2009): 895–909.

22 Xiaoli Ni, Hong Yan, Silu Chen, and Zhengwen Liu, "Factors influencing Internet addiction in a sample of freshmen university students in China," *CyberPsychology & Behavior* 12, no. 3 (2009): 327–30.

23 Sabine M. Grüesser, R. Thalemann, and M. D. Griffiths, "Excessive computer game playing: Evidence for addiction and aggression?," *CyberPsychology & Behavior* 10, no. 2 (2007): 290–92.

24 Chien-Hsin Lin, Shong-Lin Lin, and Chin-Pi Wu, "The effects of parental monitoring and leisure boredom on adolescents' internet addiction," *Adolescence* 44, no. 176 (2009): 993–1004.

25 Georgios Kormas, Elena Critselis, Mari Janikian, Dimitrios Kafetzis, and Artemis Tsitsika, "Risk factors and psychosocial characteristics of potential problematic and problematic Internet use among adolescents: A cross-sectional study," *BioMed Central Public Health* 11, research article 595 (2011): 1–8.

26 Christos C. Frangos, Constantinos C. Frangos, and Ioannis Sotiropoulos, "Problematic Internet use among Greek university students: An ordinal logistic regression with risk factors of negative psychological beliefs, pornographic sites, and online games," *Cyberpsychology, Behavior, and Social Networking* 14, no. 1–2 (2011): 51–58.

Douglas Gentile, "Pathological video-game use among youth ages 8 to 18: A National Study," *Psychological Science* 20, no. 5 (2009): 594–602.

Georgios Kormas, Elena Critselis, Mari Janikian, Dimitrios Kafetzis, and Artemis Tsitsika, "Risk factors and psychosocial characteristics of potential problematic and problematic Internet use among adolescents: A cross-sectional study," *BioMed Central Public Health* 11, research article 595 (2011): 1–8.

Lawrence T. Lam, Zi-wen Peng, Jin-cheng Mai, Jin Jing, "Factors associated with Internet addiction among adolescents," *CyberPsychology & Behavior* 12, no. 5 (2009): 551–55.

Min-Pei Lin, Huei-Chen Ko, and Jo Yung-Wei Wu, "Prevalence and psychosocial risk factors associated with Internet addiction in a nationally representative sample of college students in Taiwan," *CyberPsychology, Behavior, and Social Networking* 14, no. 12 (2011): 741–46.

Cheng-Fang Yen, Chih-Hung Ko, Ju-Yu Yen, Yu-Ping Chang, and Chung-Ping Cheng, "Multi-dimensional discriminative factors for Internet addiction among adolescents regarding gender and age," *Psychiatry and Clinical Neurosciences* 63, no. 3 (2009): 357–64.

Janet Morahan-Martin and Phyllis Schumacher, "Incidence and correlates of pathological internet use among college students," *Computers in Human Behavior* 16, no. 1 (2000): 13–29.

Roberto Poli and Emilia Agrimi, "Internet addiction disorder: Prevalence in an Italian student population," *Nordic Journal of Psychiatry* 66, no. 1 (2012): 55–59.

Hsing Fang Tsai, Shu Hui Cheng, Tzung Lieh Yeh, Chi-Chen Shih, Kao Ching Chen, Yi Ching Yang, and Yen Kuang Yang, "The risk factors of Internet addiction—A survey of university freshmen," *Psychiatry Research* 167, no. 3 (2009): 294–99.

Xin-Qiao Zhang, Yue-Qin Huang, Xiao-Min Luo, and Zhao-Rui Liu, "A cross-sectional study of Internet addiction disorder in high school students in Beijing," *Chinese Mental Health Journal* 23, no. 10 (2009): 748–51.

27 Giovanni Ferraro, Barbara Caci, Antonella D'Amico, and Marie Di Blasi, "Internet addiction disorder: An Italian Study," *CyberPsychology & Behavior* 10, no. 2 (2007): 170–75.

Richard L. Gilbert, Nora A. Murphy, and Talisa McNally, "Addiction to the 3-dimensional internet: Estimated prevalence and relationship to real world addictions," *Addiction Research and Theory* 19, no. 4 (2011): 380–90.

Huanhuan Li, Jiaqi Wang, and Li Wang, "A survey on the generalized problematic Internet use in Chinese college students and its relations to stressful life events and coping style," *International Journal of Mental Health and Addiction* 7, no. 2 (2009): 333–46.

Chien-Hsin Lin, Shong-Lin Lin, and Chin-Pi Wu, "The effects of parental monitoring and leisure boredom on adolescents' internet addiction," *Adolescence* 44, no. 176 (2009): 993–1004.

Xiaoli Ni, Hong Yan, Silu Chen, and Zhengwen Liu, "Factors influencing Internet addiction in a sample of freshmen university students in China," *CyberPsychology & Behavior* 12, no. 3 (2009): 327–30.

Soo Kyung Park, Jae Yop Kim, and Choon Bum Cho, "Prevalence of Internet addiction and correlations with family factors among south Korean adolescents," *Adolescence* 43, no. 172 (2008): 895–909.

Hui Wang, Xiaolan Zhou, Ciyong Lu, Jie Wu, Xueqing Deng, and Lingyao Hong, "Problematic Internet use in high school students in Guangdong province, China," *PLoS ONE* 6, no. 5 (2011): e19660.

28 Kimberly S. Young, "Internet addiction: The emergence of a new clinical disorder," *CyberPsychology and Behavior* 1, no. 3 (1998): 237–44.

29 Sverre Ole Drønen, "New research about Facebook addiction." http://www.uib.no/news/nyheter/2012/05/new-research-about-facebook-addiction (accessed October 3, 2012).

30 Christos C. Frangos, Constantinos C. Frangos, and Ioannis Sotiropoulos, "Problematic Internet use among Greek university students: An ordinal logistic regression with risk factors of negative psychological beliefs, pornographic sites, and online games," *Cyberpsychology, Behavior, and Social Networking* 14, nos. 1-2 (2011): 51–58.

31 Chien-Hsin Lin, Shong-Lin Lin, and Chin-Pi Wu, "The effects of parental monitoring and leisure boredom on adolescents' internet addiction," *Adolescence* 44, no. 176 (2009): 993–1004.

32 Nazir S. Hawi, "Internet addiction among adolescents in Lebanon," *Computers in Human Behavior* 28, no. 3 (2012): 1044–53.

33 Kenneth Blum, Eliot Gardner, Marlene Oscar-Berman, and Mark Gold, "'Liking' and 'wanting' linked to reward deficiency syndrome (RDS): Hypothesizing differential responsivity in brain reward circuitry," *Current Pharmaceutical Design* 18 (2012): 113–18.

34 Ibid.

35 Chih-Hung Ko, Gin-Chung Liu, Sigmund Hsiao, Ju-Yu Yen, Ming-Jen Yang, Wei-Chen Lin, Cheng-Fang Yen, and Cheng-Sheng Chen, "Brain activities associated with gaming urge of online gaming addiction," *Journal of Psychiatric Research* 43, no. 7 (2009): 739–47.

36 Lawrence T. Lam, Zi-wen Peng, Jin-cheng Mai, Jin Jing, "Factors associated with Internet addiction among adolescents," *CyberPsychology & Behavior* 12, no. 5 (2009): 551–55.

37 Ibid.

38 Douglas Gentile, "Pathological video-game use among youth ages 8 to 18: A National Study," *Psychological Science* 20, no. 5 (2009): 594–602.

39 Hui Wang, Xiaolan Zhou, Ciyong Lu, Jie Wu, Xueqing Deng, and Lingyao Hong, "Problematic Internet use in high school students in Guangdong province, China," *PLoS ONE* 6, no. 5 (2011): e19660.

40 Ibid.

41 Huanhuan Li, Jiaqi Wang, and Li Wang, "A survey on the generalized problematic Internet use in Chinese college students and its relations to stressful life events and coping style," *International Journal of Mental Health and Addiction* 7, no. 2 (2009): 333–46.

42 Ibid.

43 Janet Morahan-Martin and Phyllis Schumacher, "Incidence and correlates of pathological internet use among college students," *Computers in Human Behavior* 16, no. 1 (2000): 13–29.

44 Kanwal Nalwa and Archana Preet Anand, "Internet addiction in students: A cause of concern," *CyberPsychology & Behavior* 6, no. 6 (2003): 653–56.

45 Xiaoli Ni, Hong Yan, Silu Chen, and Zhengwen Liu, "Factors influencing Internet addiction in a sample of freshmen university students in China," *CyberPsychology & Behavior* 12, no. 3 (2009): 327–30.

46 Xin Chen, Feng-Hua Li, Li-Liang Long, et al., "Prospective study on the relationship between social support and Internet addiction," *Chinese Mental Health Journal* 4 (2007).

47 Robert Kraut, Michael Patterson, Vicki Lundmark, Sara Kiesler, Tridas Mukophadhyay, and William Scherlis, "Internet paradox: A social technology that reduces social involvement and psychological well-being," *American Psychologist* 53, no. 9 (1998): 1017–31.

48 Chih-Hung Ko, Ju-Yu Yen, Cheng-Fang Yen, Cheng-Sheng, Chen, and C. C. Chen "The association between Internet addiction and psychiatric disorder: A review of the literature," *European Psychiatry* 27, no. 1 (2012): 1–8.

Aviv Weinstein and Michel Lejoyeux, "Internet addiction or excessive Internet use," *The American Journal of Drug and Alcohol Abuse* 36, no. 5 (2010): 277–83.

Min-Pei Lin, Huei-Chen Ko, and Jo Yung-Wei Wu, "Prevalence and psychosocial risk factors associated with Internet addiction in a nationally representative sample of college students in Taiwan," *CyberPsychology, Behavior, and Social Networking* 14, no. 12 (2011): 741–46.

49 Ibid.

50 Cheng-Fang Yen, Chih-Hung Ko, Ju-Yu Yen, Yu-Ping Chang, and Chung-Ping Cheng, "Multi-dimensional discriminative factors for Internet addiction

among adolescents regarding gender and age," *Psychiatry and Clinical Neurosciences* 63, no. 3 (2009): 357–64.

51 Jee Hyun Ha, Hee Jeong Yoo, In Hee Cho, Bumsu Chin, Dongkeun Shin, and Ji Hyeon Kim, "Psychiatric comorbidity assessed in Korean children and adolescents who screen positive for Internet Addiction," *Journal of Clinical Psychiatry* 67, no. 5 (2006): 821–26.

52 Erick Messias, Juan Castro, Anil Saini, Manzoor Usman, Dale Peeples, "Sadness, suicide, and their association with video game and internet overuse among teens: Results from the Youth Risk Behavior Survey 2007 and 2009," *Suicide and Life-Threatening Behavior* 41, no. 3 (2011): 307–15.

53 Chih-Hung Ko, Ju-Yu Yen, Cheng-Fang Yen, Cheng-Sheng, Chen, and C. C. Chen, "The association between Internet addiction and psychiatric disorder: A review of the literature," *European Psychiatry* 27, no. 1 (2012): 1–8.

54 Ibid.

55 Ibid.

56 Margaret D. Weiss, Susan Baier, Blake A. Allan, Kelly Saran, and Heidi Schibuk, "The screens culture: Impact on ADHD," *ADHD Attention Deficit and Hyperactivity Disorders* 3, no. 4 (2011): 327–34.

57 Ju-Yu Yen, Cheng-Fang Yen, Cheng-Sheng Chen, Tze-Chun Tang, and Chih-Hung Ko, "The association between adult ADHD symptoms and Internet addiction among college students: The gender difference," *CyberPsychology & Behavior* 12, no. 2 (2009): 187–91.

58 Hee-Jeong Yoo, Surl-Churl Cho, Jihyun Ha, Sook-Kyung Yune, Seog-Ju Kim, Jaeuk Hwang, Ain Chung, Young-Hoon Sung, In-Kyoon Lyoo, "Attention deficit hyperactivity symptoms and Internet addiction," *Psychiatry and Clinical Neurosciences* 58, no. 5 (2004): 487–94.

59 Chih-Hung Ko, Ju-Yu Yen, Cheng-Fang Yen, Cheng-Sheng Chen, and C. C. Chen, "The association between Internet addiction and psychiatric disorder: A review of the literature," *European Psychiatry* 27, no. 1 (2012): 1–8.

60 Ibid.

61 Ibid.

62 Chien-Hsin Lin, Shong-Lin Lin, and Chin-Pi Wu, "The effects of parental monitoring and leisure boredom on adolescents' Internet addiction," *Adolescence* 44, no. 176 (2009): 993–1004.

63 Cheng-Fang Yen, Chih-Hung Ko, Ju-Yu Yen, Yu-Ping Chang, and Chung-Ping Cheng, "Multi-dimensional discriminative factors for Internet addiction among adolescents regarding gender and age," *Psychiatry and Clinical Neurosciences* 63, no. 3 (2009): 357–64.

64 Hui Wang, Xiaolan Zhou, Ciyong Lu, Jie Wu, Xueqing Deng, and Lingyao Hong, "Problematic Internet Use in High School Students in Guangdong Province, China," *PLoS ONE* 6, no. 5 (2011): e19660.

65 Lawrence T. Lam, Zi-wen Peng, Jin-cheng Mai, Jin Jing, "Factors associated with Internet addiction among adolescents," *CyberPsychology & Behavior* 12, no. 5 (2009): 551–55.

66 Soo Kyung Park, Jae Yop Kim, and Choon Bum Cho, "Prevalence of Internet addiction and correlations with family factors among south Korean adolescents," *Adolescence* 43, no. 172 (2008): 895–909.

67 Xin-Qiao Zhang, Yue-Qin Huang, Xiao-Min Luo, and Zhao-Rui Liu, "A cross-sectional study of Internet addiction disorder in high school students in Beijing," *Chinese Mental Health Journal* 23, no. 10 (2009): 748–51.

68 Xiaoli Ni, Hong Yan, Silu Chen, and Zhengwen Liu, "Factors influencing Internet addiction in a sample of freshmen university students in China," *CyberPsychology & Behavior* 12, no. 3 (2009): 327–30.

69 Xin-Qiao Zhang, Yue-Qin Huang, Xiao-Min Luo, and Zhao-Rui Liu, "A cross-sectional study of Internet addiction disorder in high school students in Beijing," *Chinese Mental Health Journal* 23, no. 10 (2009): 748–51.

70 Georgios Kormas, Elena Critselis, Mari Janikian, Dimitrios Kafetzis, and Artemis Tsitsika, "Risk factors and psychosocial characteristics of potential problematic and problematic Internet use among adolescents: A cross-sectional study," *BioMed Central Public Health* 11, research article 595 (2011): 1–8.

71 Chih-Hung Ko, Huang-Chi Lin, Ju-Yu Yen, Cheng-Fang Yen, and Ming-Jen Yang, "Factors predictive for incidence and remission of Internet addiction in young adolescents: A prospective study," *CyberPsychology and Behavior* 10, no. 4 (2007): 545-51.

72 Hui Wang, Xiaolan Zhou, Ciyong Lu, Jie Wu, Xueqing Deng, and Lingyao Hong, "Problematic Internet use in high school students in Guangdong province, China," *PLoS ONE* 6, no. 5 (2011): e19660.

73 Shi-jie Zhou, Zhi-hong Tang, Yang Peng, "Internet-related behavior characteristics of adolescents with Internet addiction," *Chinese Journal of Clinical Psychology* 17, no. 2 (2009): 151–53.

74 Richard L. Gilbert, Nora A. Murphy, and Talisa McNally, "Addiction to the 3-dimensional internet: Estimated prevalence and relationship to real world addictions," *Addiction Research and Theory* 19, no. 4 (2011): 380–90.

75 Kimberly S. Young, "Internet addiction: The emergence of a new clinical disorder." *CyberPsychology and Behavior* 1, no. 3 (1998): 237–44.

76 Richard L. Gilbert, Nora A. Murphy, and Talisa McNally, "Addiction to the 3-dimensional internet: Estimated prevalence and relationship to real world addictions," *Addiction Research and Theory* 19, no. 4 (2011): 380–90.

77 Ibid.

78 Douglas Gentile, "Pathological video-game use among youth ages 8 to 18: A national study," *Psychological Science* 20, no. 5 (2009): 594–602.

79 Shi-jie Zhou, Zhi-hong Tang, Yang Peng, "Internet-related behavior characteristics of adolescents with Internet addiction," *Chinese Journal of Clinical Psychology* 17, no. 2 (2009): 151–53.

80 Hui Wang, Xiaolan Zhou, Ciyong Lu, Jie Wu, Xueqing Deng, and Lingyao Hong, "Problematic Internet use in high school students in Guangdong province, China," *PLoS ONE* 6, no. 5 (2011): e19660.

81 Min-Pei Lin, Huei-Chen Ko, and Jo Yung-Wei Wu, "Prevalence and psychosocial risk factors associated with Internet addiction in a nationally representative sample of college students in Taiwan," *CyberPsychology, Behavior, and Social Networking* 14, no. 12 (2011): 741–46.

82 Dimitri A. Christakis and Megan A. Moreno, "Trapped in the net: Will Internet addiction become a 21st-century epidemic?," *Archives of Pediatrics and Adolescent Medicine* 163, no. 10 (2009): 959–60.

83 Min-Pei Lin, Huei-Chen Ko, and Jo Yung-Wei Wu, "Prevalence and psychosocial risk factors associated with Internet addiction in a nationally representative sample of college students in Taiwan," *CyberPsychology, Behavior, and Social Networking* 14, no. 12 (2011): 744.

84 Ronald Pies, "Should DSM-V designate "Internet addiction" a mental disorder?" *Psychiatry* 6, no. 2 (2009): 31–37.

85 Ibid.

86 American Psychiatric Association, "*DSM-5 Development.*" http://www.dsm5.org/proposedrevision/Pages/proposedrevision.aspx?rid=573 (accessed October 3, 2012).

87 Ibid.

88 Nathan A. Shapira, Mary C. Lessig, Toby D. Goldsmith, Steven T. Szabo,

Martin Lazoritz, Mark S. Gold, and Dan J. Stein, "Problematic internet use: Proposed classification and diagnostic criteria," *Depression and Anxiety* 17, no. 4 (2003): 207–16.

89 Kimberly S. Young, "CBT-IA: The first treatment model for Internet addiction," *Journal of Cognitive Psychotherapy: An International Quarterly* 25, no. 4 (2011): 304–12.

90 G. J. Meerkerk, R. J. J. M. Van Den Eijnden, A. A Vermulst, and H. F. L. Garretsen, "The Compulsive Internet Use Scale (CIUS): Some psychometric properties," *CyberPsychology & Behavior* 12, no. 1 (2009): 1–6.

91 Janet Morahan-Martin and Phyllis Schumacher, "Incidence and correlates of pathological internet use among college students," *Computers in Human Behavior* 16, no. 1 (2000): 13–29.

92 Douglas A. Gentile, "Pathological video game use among youth 8 to 18: A national study," *Psychological Science* 20, no. 6 (2009): 785.

93 Martha Shaw and Donald W. Black, "Internet addiction: Definition, assessment, epidemiology and clinical management," *CNS Drugs* 22, no. 5 (2008): 353–65.

94 Chih-Hung Ko, Ju-Yu Yen, Cheng-Fang Yen, Cheng-Sheng Chen, and C. C. Chen, "The association between Internet addiction and psychiatric disorder: A review of the literature," *European Psychiatry* 27 (2012): 1–8.

95 Kimberly S. Young, *Caught in the Net: How to Recognize the Signs of Internet Addiction- and a Winning Strategy for Recovery* (New York: John Wiley & Sons, Inc. 1998).

96 Georgios Kormas, Elena Critselis, Mari Janikian, Dimitrios Kafetzis, and Artemis Tsitsika, "Risk factors and psychosocial characteristics of potential problematic and problematic Internet use among adolescents: A cross-sectional study," *BioMed Central Public Health* 11, research article 595 (2011): 1–8.

97 Chih-Hung Ko, Gin-Chung Liu, Sigmund Hsiao, Ju-Yu Yen, Ming-Jen Yang, Wei-Chen Lin, Cheng-Fang Yen, and Cheng-Sheng Chen, "Brain activities associated with gaming urge of online gaming addiction," *Journal of Psychiatric Research* 43, no. 7 (2009): 739–47.

98 Kimberly S. Young, "Internet sex addiction: Risk factors, stages of development, and treatment," *American Behavioral Scientist* 52, no. 21 (2008): 21–37.

99 Christiano Nabuco de Abreu and Dora Sampaio Goes, "Psychotherapy for internet addiction," in *Internet Addiction: A Handbook and Guide to Evaluation and Treatment* ed. by Kimberly S. Young and Christiano Nabuco de Abreu (Hoboken, NJ: John Wiley & Sons, Inc., 2011), 155–171.

100 Ibid.

101 Ibid.

102 Kimberly S. Young, "Internet sex addiction: Risk factors, stages of development, and treatment," *American Behavioral Scientist* 52, no. 21 (2008): 21–37.

103 Kimberly S. Young, "CBT-IA: The first treatment model for Internet addiction," *Journal of Cognitive Psychotherapy: An International Quarterly* 25, no. 4 (2011): 304–12.

104 Ibid.

105 Lukas Blinka and David Smahel, "Addiction to online role-playing games," in *Internet Addiction: A Handbook and Guide to Evaluation and Treatment*, ed. by Kimberly S. Young and Christiano Nabuco de Abreu (Hoboken, NJ: John Wiley & Sons, Inc., 2011), 73–90.

106 Ibid.

107 Huanhuan Li, Jiaqi Wang, and Li Wang, "A survey on the generalized problematic Internet use in Chinese college students and its relations to stressful life events and coping style," *International Journal of Mental Health and Addiction* 7, no. 2 (2009): 333–46.

108 Christiano Nabuco de Abreu and Dora Sampaio Goes, "Psychotherapy for internet addiction," in *Internet Addiction: A Handbook and Guide to Evaluation and Treatment*, ed. by Kimberly S. Young and Christiano Nabuco de Abreu (Hoboken, NJ: John Wiley & Sons, Inc., 2011), 155–71.

109 Ibid.

110 Ibid.

111 Doug Hyun Han, Sun Mi Kim, Young Sik Lee, and Perry F. Renshaw, "The effect of family therapy on the changes in the severity of on-line game play and brain activity in adolescents with on-line game addiction," *Psychiatry Research: Neuroimaging* 202, no. 2 (2012): 126–31.

112 Xin Zhong, Si Zu, Sha Sha, Ran Tao, Chongsi Zhao, Fengchi Yang, Mei Li, and Peng Sha, "The effect of a family-based intervention model on Internet-addicted Chinese adolescents," *Social Behavior and Personality* 39, no. 8 (2011): 1021–34.

113 Ibid.

114 Kimberly Young, "Understanding online gaming addiction and treatment issues for adolescents," *The American Journal of Family Therapy* 37 (2009): 355–72.

115 Keith W. Beard, "Working with adolescents addicted to the Internet," in *Internet Addiction: A Handbook and Guide to Evaluation and Treatment,* ed. by Kimberly S. Young and Christiano Nabuco de Abreu (Hoboken, NJ: John Wiley & Sons, Inc., 2011), 173–89.

116 Ibid.

117 Judith Landau, James Garrett, and Robert Webb, "Assisting a concerned person to motivate someone experiencing cybersex into treatment: Application of invitational intervention: The ARISE model to cybersex," *Journal of Marital and Family Therapy* 34, no. 4 (2008): 498–511.

118 Raymond M. Bergner and Ana J. Bridges, "The significance of heavy pornography involvement for romantic partners: Research and clinical implications," *Journal of Sex & Marital Therapy* 28 (2002): 193–206.

119 Ibid.

120 Jeffrey J. Ford, Jared A. Durtschi, and Darrell L. Franklin, "Structural therapy with a couple battling pornography addiction," *The American Journal of Family Therapy* 40 (2012): 336–48.

Glossary

A

Abstinence A voluntary choice to not engage in a particular behavior. In the case of addiction, the behavior can include an activity such as sex or gambling, or it may include the taking of a substance such as alcohol or other drug.

Action gambler A gambler who chooses games requiring skill or knowledge. Preferred games include poker, dice, craps, sports betting, or the stock market, and are highly competitive.

Addiction The compulsive attraction or a pathological attachment to a substance, normally to a drug.

Amino acids Organic compounds that combine to form proteins.

Amygdalae A part of the brain involved in sexual response, anger, aggression, and fear.

Anterior cingulate cortex A fibrous collar shaped bundle that relays neural signals between the right and left hemispheres of the brain, regulating blood pressure, heart rate, and plays a key role in decision-making, reward anticipation and emotions.

Axons The single process of a nerve cell that conducts nerve impulses away from the cell body and its remaining processes. The other type is the dendrite.

B

Basal ganglia A group of structures located deep within the brain that regulates movement.

Bulimarexia Eating disorder characterized by the alternation between an aversion to, and an abnormal craving for, food.

C

Compulsive gamblers Term used by laypersons to describe gamblers whose behavior meets the diagnostic criteria of a pathological gambler.

Compulsivity The performance of repetitive behaviors with the goal of reducing or preventing anxiety or distress; the goal is not to provide pleasure or gratification.

Cross tolerance Use of one addiction to otherwise moderate, relieve, or avoid withdrawal from another addiction.

Current comorbidity The occurrence of two or more disorders at the same time. For example, someone may be a pathological gambler, suffer from depression or AD/HD, and have other compulsions or addictions.

D

Dendrite A type of branching protoplasmic processes of the nerve cell. The other type is the axon.

Desperation phase Third phase of gambling where the gambler experiences the onset of health problems, deterioration of relationships, legal problems, and hopelessness. Clinging to the hope that a big win is imminent the gambler may steal, write bad checks, or commit other crimes to finance gambling.

Disordered gambling A term often used to describe compulsive or problem gambling.

Down-regulation A process where a cell decreases a cellular component in response to an external variable. See also *neuronal tolerance.*

E

Effector cells A nerve ending that carries impulses to a muscle, gland, or organ.

Ego-dystonic The nature or tendency to seek the avoidance of harm.

Ego-systonic The nature or tendency to seek the attainment of pleasure.

Endocannabinoids Naturally occurring substances in the body that activate the cannabinoid receptors.

Escape gambler A gambler who chooses games that do not require skill or knowledge. Preferred games include video poker, slot machines, bingo, etc. whereby the gambler develops a "system" to try to win.

G

Glutamate The most abundant excitatory neurotransmitter in the central nervous system that is used to build proteins in the body.

H

Harm reduction A therapy where the established goal is for a gambler to learn to control or modify their gambling.

Hopeless phase Fourth and final phase of gambling where the gambler has lost all hope, is severely depressed, and may contemplate or commit suicide.

I

Impulsivity Goal-directed behavior characterized by poor judgment in the attainment of rewards where the seeking of pleasure continues despite harmful consequences.

Interneurons Nerve cells within the central nervous system that act as links between motor neurons and sensory neurons.

Ionotropic Affecting the force of muscular contractions.

K

Kainate Comes from kainic acid (marine acid) present in some seaweed. Specialized receptors use kainite, which responds to glutamate.

L

Level 0 gambling Refers to individuals who have never gambled.

Level 1 gambling Refers to individuals who are social or recreational gamblers.

Level 2 gambling Refers to individuals who are at-risk gamblers and who are experiencing some problems associated with their gambling.

Level 3 gambling Refers to individuals who are pathological gamblers and meet the established criteria for pathological gambling.

Level One sexual behaviors Sexual behaviors that are not uncommon and considered normal and usually victimless to most nonsexual addicts.

Level Three sexual behaviors Sexual behaviors considered forms of serious victimization such as rape, incest, and sexual molestation. Force or threat of violence may play a factor.

Level Two sexual behaviors Sexual behaviors considered mild or non-violent forms of "victimization" such as voyeurism, exhibitionism, or obscene phone calls.

Lifetime comorbidity The occurrence of two, or more, disorders over the course of a person's lifetime. The disorders are not experienced concurrently.

Locus coeruleus A nucleus in the brain stem that controls physical response to panic and stress.

Losing phase The second phase of gambling where the gambler becomes preoccupied. Phase is characterized by the need to place larger bets and to chase losses.

M

Mesolimbic dopamine system (MDS) A pathway in the brain in which dopamine is carried from one part of the brain to another. It is associated with movement, compulsion and preservation, as well as pleasure and reward.

Metabotropic Relating to a glutamate receptor that triggers increased production of cell messengers.

N

Neurons Also called nerve cells, neurons are excitable cells located in the nervous system that process and transmit information. They are the core of the brain and spinal cord.

Neuropeptides Signaling molecules used by neurons to communicate with each other.

Neurotransmitters Chemicals in the brain that transmit nerve impulses across a synapse.

Norepinephrine A stress hormone affecting the parts of the brain concerned with attention and responding actions.

Nucleus accumbens A collection of neurons in the brain thought to be responsible for reward, pleasure, fear, laughter, depression, and addiction.

Nucleus coeruleus Located in the brainstem, it is involved with physical response to panic and stress.

P

Paraphilia Sometimes referred to as sexual deviation. It is a psychosexual disorder whereby someone fantasizes and/or engages in sex with inanimate objects, a non-consenting partner, the infliction of pain or humiliation on a sex partner or oneself.

Pathological Behavior that may be caused by or related to a disease; the behavior is compulsive, addictive, or maladaptive in nature. Examples include pathological liar or pathological gambler.

Pathological gambler Individuals whose gambling behavior meets at least five of the ten criteria as determined by the *Diagnostic and Statistical Manual of the American Psychological Association Fourth Edition Text Revision (DSM IV-TR)*.

Pathways Model Maintains that multiple factors cause problem gambling; factors include behavioral conditioning, emotional vulnerability, and antisocial or impulsive personality traits.

Pons Located on the brain stem between the two hemispheres of the brain, it coordinates communications between the spheres.

Prefrontal cortex An area of the brain responsible for planning for the future and taking action. It is also responsible for dopamine pathways and plays a role in addiction and pleasure.

Problem gambler Individual whose gambling behavior meets at least three of the ten diagnostic criteria for gambling addiction as determined by the *Diagnostic and Statistical Manual of the American Psychological Association Fourth Edition Text Revision (DSM IV-TR)*.

Problem gambling Term reserved for those individuals whose behavior meets at least three of the *DSM-IV-TR* diagnostic criteria for gambling addiction.

R

Raphe nucleus A cluster of cells found in the brain stem primarily responsible for releasing serotonin to the rest of the brain.

Receptor A structural protein molecule within the cytoplasm or on the cell surface, that binds to a specific hormone, drug, antigen, or neurotransmitter.

Reuptake The process of re-absorption of a neurotransmitter after it has performed its function of transmitting a neural (nerve) impulse.

S

Subcortical Refers to the subcortex, which is immediately below the cerebral cortex.

Substantia nigra A brain structure, which plays a vital role in both addiction and reward.

Synapse The functional membrane-to-membrane contact of a nerve cell with another nerve cell, a sensory receptor cell, or a muscle or gland (effector) cell.

Synaptic cleft The small gap between an axon terminal and a nearby cell.

T

Telescoping A rapid progression into compulsive gambling found to be more common in women than in men. Men may begin gambling earlier in life than women, but men seem to progress at a much slower rate.

U

u-opioid receptor antagonist A drug used to treat drug and alcohol dependence that shows promise in the treatment of other addictions such as gambling.

Upregulation An increase in the number of receptors on the surface of target cells making the cells more sensitive to a hormone.

V

Ventral pallidum A structure within the basal ganglia of the brain involved in emotions, behavior, and motivation; receives dopamine from the ventral tegmental area and addictive substances that facilitate a dopamine release in this area of the brain.

Ventral tegmental area (VTA) A portion or part of the midbrain stem consisting of dopamine pathways; it is responsible for pleasure.

W

Winning phase Initial phase of gambling when an individual finds the activity fun, exciting, or as a way to escape the stressors of life; this phase is typically characterized by winning large sums of money. In this phase players may have "beginner's luck," which ultimately leads to betting ever-larger sums of money with or without an increase in frequency.

Bibliography

Adams, Kenneth M., and Donald W. Robinson. "Shame reduction, affect regulation, and sexual boundary development: Essential building blocks of sexual addiction treatment." *Sexual Addiction & Compulsivity* 8, no. 1 (2001): 23–44.

Albrecht, Ulrike, Nina E. Kirschner, and Sabine M. Grüsser. "Diagnostic instruments for behavioural addiction: An overview." *GMS Psycho-Social-Medicine* 4, doc. 11 (2007): 1–11.

Amen, Daniel G., Kristen Willeumier, and Robert Johnson. "The clinical utility of brain SPECT imaging in process addictions." *Journal of Psychoactive Drugs* 44, no. 1 (2012): 18–26.

American Psychiatric Association, *Diagnostic and Statistical Manual of Mental Disorders*: 3rd ed. Washington DC: American Psychiatric Association, 1980.

American Psychiatric Association, *Diagnostic and Statistical Manual of Mental Disorders:* 4th ed. Washington, DC: American Psychiatric Association, 1994.

American Psychiatric Association, *Diagnostic and Statistical Manual of Mental Disorders*: 4th ed., text rev., Washington, DC, American Psychiatric Association, 2000.

Anderson, Drew A., Jennifer D. Lundgren, Jennifer R. Shapiro, and Carrie A. Paulosky. "Assessment of eating disorders: Review and recommendations for clinical use." *Behavior Modification* 28, no. 6 (2004): 763–82.

Anderson, Drew A., Matthew P. Martens, and M. Dolores Cimini. "Do female college students who purge report greater alcohol use and negative alcohol-related consequences?" *International Journal of Eating Disorders* 37, no. 1 (2005): 65–68.

Baker, Jessica H., Karen S. Mitchell, Michael C. Neale, and Kenneth S. Kendler. "Eating disorder symptomatology and substance use disorders: Prevalence and shared risk in a population-based twin sample." *International Journal of Eating Disorders* 43, no. 7 (2010): 648–58.

Baker, Jessica H., Suzanne E. Mazzeo, and Kenneth S. Kendler. "Association between broadly defined bulimia nervosa and drug use disorders: Common genetic and environmental influences." *International Journal of Eating Disorders* 40, no. 8 (2007): 673–78.

Barry, Kristen L., and Michael F. Fleming. "Family cohesion, expressiveness, and conflict in alcoholic families." *British Journal of Addiction* 85, no. 1 (1990): 81–87.

Baylé, Franck J., Hervé Caci, Bruno Millet, Sami Richa, and Jean-Pierre Olié. "Psychopathology and comorbidity of psychiatric disorders in patients with kleptomania." *American Journal of Psychiatry* 160, no. 8 (2003): 1509–13.

Beard, Keith W. "Internet addiction: A review of current assessment techniques and potential assessment questions." *CyberPsychology & Behavior* 8, no. 1, (2005): 7–14.

Beard, Keith W. "Working with adolescents addicted to the internet." In *Internet Addiction: A Handbook and Guide to Evaluation and Treatment*, edited by Kimberly S. Young and Christiano Nabuco de Abreu. Hoboken, NJ: John Wiley & Sons, Inc., 2011.

Beary, M. D., J. H. Lacey, and Julius Merry. "Alcoholism and eating disorders in women of fertile age." *British Journal of Addiction* 81, no. 5 (1986): 685–89.

Bello, Nicholas T., and Andras Hajnal. "Dopamine and binge eating behaviors." *Pharmacology, Biochemistry and Behavior* 97, no. 1 (2010): 25–33.

Black, David W., Laura L. D. Kehrberg, Denise L. Flumerfelt, and Steven S. Schlosser. "Characteristics of 36 subjects reporting compulsive sexual behavior." *American Journal of Psychiatry* 154, no. 2 (1997): 243–50.

Blanco, Carlos, Analucia A. Alegria, Nancy M. Petry, Jon E. Grant, H. Blair Simpson, Shang- Min Liu, Bridget F. Grant, and Deborah S. Hasin. "Prevalence and correlates of fire-setting in the United States: Results from the National Epidemiological Survey on Alcohol and Related Conditions (NESARC)." *Journal of Clinical Psychiatry* 71, no. 9 (2010): 1218–25.

Blanco, Carlos, Angela Ibáñez, Jerónimo Sáiz-Ruiz, Carmen Blanco-Jerez, and Edward V. Nunes. "Epidemiology, pathophysiology, and treatment of pathological gambling." *CNS Drugs* 13, no. 6 (2000): 397–407.

Blanco, Carlos, Jon Grant, Nancy M. Petry, H. Blair Simpson, Analucia A. Alegria, Shang-Min Liu, and Deborah Hasin. "Prevalence and correlates of shoplifting in the United States: Results from the National Epidemiological Survey on Alcohol and Related Conditions (NESARC)." *American Journal of Psychiatry* 165, no. 7 (2008): 905–13.

Blankenship, Richard, and Mark Laaser. "Sexual addiction and ADHD: Is there a connection?" *Sexual Addiction & Compulsivity* 11 (2004): 7–20.

Blaszczynski, Alex, and Eimear Farrell. "A case series of 44 completed gambling-related suicides." *Journal of Gambling Studies* 14, no. 2 (1998): 93–109.

Blinder, Barton J., Edward J. Cumella, and Visant A. Sanathara. "Psychiatric comorbidities of female inpatients with eating disorders." *Psychosomatic Medicine* 68 (2006): 454–62.

Blinka, Lukas, and David Smahel. "Addiction to online role-playing games." In *Internet Addiction: A Handbook and Guide to Evaluation and Treatment*, edited by Kimberly S. Young and Christiano Nabuco de Abreu. Hoboken, NJ: John Wiley & Sons, Inc., 2011.

Blum, Kenneth, Amanda L. C. Chen, Thomas J. H. Chen, Eric R. Braverman, Jeffrey Reinking, Seth H. Blum, Kimberly Cassel, Bernard W. Downs, Roger L. Waite, Lonna Williams, Thomas J. Prihoda, Mallory M. Kerner, Tomas Palomo, David E. Comings, Howard Tung, Patrick Rhodes, and Marlene Oscar-Berman. "Activation instead of blocking mesolimbic dopaminergic reward circuitry is a preferred modality in the long term treatment of reward deficiency syndrome (RDS): a commentary." *Theoretical Biology and Medical Modeling* 5, no. 24 (2008): 5–24.

Blum, Kenneth, Eliot Gardner, Marlene Oscar-Berman, and Mark Gold. "'Liking' and 'wanting' linked to reward deficiency syndrome (RDS): Hypothesizing differential responsivity in brain reward circuitry." *Current Pharmaceutical Design* 17 (2011): 1–5.

Bonfà, F., S. Cabrini, M. Avanzi, O. Bettinardi, R. Spotti, and E. Uber. "Treatment dropout in drug-addicted women: Are eating disorders implicated?" *Eating and Weight Disorders* 13, no. 2 (2008): 81–86.

Boughton, Roberta, and Olesya Falenchuk. "Vulnerability and comorbidity factors of female problem gambling." *Journal of Gambling Studies* 23, no. 3 (2007): 323–34.

Brecht, Mary-Lynn, Ann O'Brien, Christina von Mayrhauser, and M. Douglas Anglin. "Methamphetamine use behaviors and gender differences." *Addictive Behaviors* 29, issue 1 (2004): 89–106.

Bulik, Cynthia M. "Alcohol use and depression in women with bulimia." *American Journal of Drug and Alcohol Abuse* 13, no. 3 (1987a): 343–55.

Bulik, Cynthia M. "Drug and alcohol abuse by bulimic women and their families." *American Journal of Psychiatry* 144, no. 12 (1987b): 1604–6.

Bulik, Cynthia M., and Emma C. Brinded. "The effect of food deprivation on alcohol consumption in bulimic and control women." *Addiction* 88, no. 11 (1993): 1545–51.

Bulik, Cynthia M., and Patrick F. Sullivan. "Comorbidity of bulimia and substance abuse: Perceptions of family of origin." *International Journal of Eating Disorders* 13, no. 1 (1993): 49–56.

Button, Eric J., Bhanu Chadalavada, and Robert L. Palmer. "Mortality and predictors of death in a cohort of patients presenting to an eating disorder service." *International Journal of Eating Disorders* 43, no. 5 (2010): 387–92.

Cappell, Howard, and C. Peter Herman. "Alcohol and tension reduction: A review." *Quarterly Journal of Studies on Alcohol* 33, no. 1-A (1972): 33–64.

Carnes, Patrick J. *Out of the Shadows: Understanding Sexual Addiction,* Center City, MN: Hazelden Information and Education, 2001.

Carnes, Patrick J., Brad Green, and Stefanie Carnes. "The same yet different: Refocusing the Sexual Addiction Screening Test (SAST) to reflect orientation and gender." *Sexual Addiction & Compulsivity* 17, no. 1 (2010): 7–30.

Carnes, Patrick J., Robert E. Murray, Louis Charpenter. "Bargains with chaos: Sex addicts and addiction interaction disorder." *Sexual Addiction & Compulsivity* 12 (2005): 79–120.

Carroll, M. E., C. P. France, and R. A. Meisch. "Food deprivation increases oral and intravenous drug intake in rats. *Science* 205, no. 4403 (1979): 319–21.

Cassin, Stephanie E., and Kristin M. von Ranson. "Is binge eating experienced as an addiction?" *Appetite* 49, no. 3 (2007): 687–90.

Castro-Fornieles, Josefina, J. Rosa Diaz, Javier Goti, Rosa Calvo, Laura Gonzalez, Lourdes Serrano, and Antoni Gual. "Prevalence and factors related to substance use among adolescents with eating disorders." *European Addiction Research* 16, no. 2 (2010): 61–68.

Center for Substance Abuse Treatment. *Substance Abuse Treatment for Persons With Co-Occurring Disorders.* Treatment Improvement Protocol (TIP) 42. DHHS Publication No. SMA 05-3922. Rockville, MD: U.S. Department of Health and Human Services, Public Health Service (2005).

Çepik, Asli, Zehra Arikan, Cumhar Boratav, and Erdal Lsik. "Bulimia in a male alcoholic: A symptom substitution in alcoholism." *International Journal of Eating Disorders* 17, no. 2 (1995): 201–4.

Chamberlain, Samuel R., Brian L. Odlaug, Vasileios Boulougouris, Naomi Fineberg, and Jon E. Grant. "Trichotillomania: Neurobiology and treatment." *Neuroscience and Biobehavioral Reviews* 33 (2009): 831–42.

Chamberlain, Samuel R., Lara Menzies, Barbara J. Sahakian, and Naomi A. Fineberg. "Lifting the veil on trichotillomania." *American Journal of Psychiatry* 164, no. 4 (2007): 568–74.

Chambers, R. Andrew, Jane R. Taylor, Marc N. Potenza. "Developmental neurocircuitry of motivation in adolescence: A critical period of addiction vulnerability." *American Journal of Psychiatry* 160, no. 6 (2003): 1041–52.

Chen, Xin, Feng-Hua Li, Li-Liang Long. "Prospective study on the relationship between social support and internet addiction." *Chinese Mental Health Journal* 21, no. 4 (2007): 240–43.

Christakis, Dimitri A., and Megan A. Moreno. "Trapped in the net: Will internet addiction become a 21st-century epidemic?" *Archives of Pediatrics and Adolescent* Medicine 163, no. 10 (2009): 959–60.

Ciarrocchi, Joseph W. *Counseling Problem Gamblers: A Self-Regulation Manual for Individual and Family Therapy.* San Diego: Academic Press, 2002.

Coccaro, Emil F., Royce J. Lee, and Richard J. Kavoussi. "A double-blind, randomized, placebo-controlled trial of fluoxetine in patients with intermittent explosive disorder." *Journal of Clinical Psychiatry* 70, no. 5 (2009): 653–62.

Cohen, Lisa R., Shelly F. Greenfield, Susan Gordon, Theresa Killeen, Huiping Jiang, Yulei Zhang, and Denise Hien. "Survey of eating disorder symptoms among women in treatment for substance abuse." *The American Journal on Addictions* 19, no. 3 (2010): 245–51.

Conason, A. H., A. Brunstein Klomek, and L. Sher. "Recognizing alcohol and drug abuse in patients with eating disorders." *Quarterly Journal of Medicine* 99 (2006): 335–39.

Cooper, Zafra, and Christopher Fairburn. "The eating disorder examination: A semi-structured interview for the assessment of the specific psychopathology of eating disorders." *International Journal of Eating Disorders* 6, no. 1 (1987): 1–8.

Corey, Gerald. *Theory and Practice of Counseling and Psychotherapy.* 7th ed. Belmont, CA: Brooks/Cole-Thompson Learning, 2005.

Cowan, Jennifer, and Carol Devine. "Food, eating, and weight concerns of men in recovery from substance addiction." *Appetite* 50, no. 1 (2008): 33–42.

Crockford, David N., and Nady el-Guebaly. "Psychiatric comorbidity in pathological gambling: A critical review." *Canadian Journal of Psychiatry* 43, no. 1 (1998): 43–50.

Cunningham, John A. "Little use of treatment among problem gamblers." *Psychiatric Services* 56, no. 8 (2005): 1024–25.

Curran, H. Valerie, and Katy Robjant. "Eating attitudes, weight concerns, and beliefs about drug effects in women who use ecstasy." *Journal of Psychopharmacology* 20, no. 3 (2006): 425–31.

Custer, Robert L., and Harry Milt. *When Luck Runs Out: Help for Compulsive Gamblers and Their Families.* New York: Facts on File, 1985.

Dansky, Bonnie S., Timothy D. Brewerton, and Dean G. Kilpatrick. "Comorbidity of bulimia nervosa and alcohol use disorders: Results from the National Women's Study." *International Journal of Eating Disorders* 27, no. 2 (2000): 180–90.

Dawe, Sharon, and Natalie J. Loxton. "The role of impulsivity in the development of substance use and eating disorders." *Neuroscience and Biobehavioral Reviews* 28, no. 3 (2004): 343–51.

Del Giudice, Matthew J., and Joshua Kutinsky. "Applying motivational interviewing to the treatment of sexual compulsivity and addiction." *Sexual Addiction & Compulsivity* 14, no. 4 (2001): 303–19.

Dell'Osso, Bernardo A. Carlo Altamura, Andrea Allen, Donatella Marazziti, and Eric Hollander. "Epidemiologic and clinical updates on impulse control disorders: A critical review." *European Archives of Psychiatry and Clinical Neuroscience* 256 (2006): 464–75.

Delmonico, David L., Donald Bubenzer, and John D. West. "Assessing sexual addiction with the sexual dependency inventory-revised." *Sexual Addiction & Compulsivity* 5, no. 3 (1998): 179–86.

Derevensky, Jeffrey L., and Rina Gupta. *Gambling Problems in Youth: Theoretical and Applied Perspectives.* New York: Kluwer Academic/Plenum Publishers, 2004.

Derevensky, Jeffrey L., Rina Gupta, Laurie Dickson, and Anne-Elyse Deguire. "Prevention efforts toward reducing gambling problems." In *Gambling Problems in Youth: Theoretical and Applied Perspectives,* edited by Jeffrey L. Derevensky and Rina Gupta, 211–30. New York: Kluwer Academic/Plenum Publishers, 2004.

Desai, Rani A., Paul K. Maciejewski, David J. Dausey, Barbara J. Caldarone, and Marc N. Potenza. "Health correlates of recreational gambling in older adults." *American Journal of Psychiatry* 161, no. 9 (2004): 1672–79.

Dunn, Eric C., Mary E. Larimer, and Clayton Neighbors. "Alcohol and drug-related negative consequences in college students with bulimia nervosa and binge eating disorder." *International Journal of Eating Disorders* 32, no. 2 (2002): 171–78.

Emerson, Margaret H., Ellen Glovsky, Hortensia Amaro, and Rita Nieves. "Unhealthy weight gain during treatment for alcohol and drug use in four residential programs for Latina and African American women." *Substance Use and Misuse* 4, no. 11 (2009): 1553–65.

Erickson, Carlton K. *The Science of Addiction: From Neurobiology to Treatment.* New York: W. W. Norton & Company, 2007.

Evans, Rod L., and Mark Hance. *Legalized Gambling: For and Against.* Chicago: Open Court Publishing Company, 1998.

Everitt, Barry J., and Trevor W. Robbins. "Neural systems of reinforcement for drug addiction: From actions to habits to compulsion." *Nature Neuroscience* 8 (2005): 1481–89.

Fairburn, Christopher G., and Paul J. Harrison. "Eating disorders." *Lancet* 361, no. 9355 (2003): 407–16.

Fairburn, Christopher G., and Zafra Cooper. "The Eating Disorder Examination, 12th ed." In *Binge Eating: Nature, Assessment, and Treatment,* edited by Christopher G. Fairburn and G. Terence Wilson, 317–60. New York, NY: The Guilford Press, 1993.

Ferree, Marnie C. "Females and sex addiction: Myths and diagnostic implications." *Sexual Addiction & Compulsivity* 8, nos. 3-4 (2001): 287–300.

Fisher, Gary L., and Thomas C. Harrison. *Substance Abuse: Information for School Counselors, Social Workers, Therapists, and Counselors.* 5th ed. Boston: Pearson Education, Inc., 2013.

Flood, M. "Addictive eating disorders." *Nursing Interventions for Addicted Patients* 24 (1989): 45–53.

Food and Drug Administration. (2007). *Desoxyn: Methamphetamine Hydrochloride Tablets, USP.* Med Guide. Retrieved from http://www.accessdata.fda.gov/drugsatfda_docs/label/2007/005378s026lbl.pdf.

Frank, Robert E., Mary K. Serdula, and Daniel Adame. "Weight loss and bulimic eating behavior: Changing patterns within a population of young adult women." *Southern Medical Journal* 84, no. 4 (1991): 457–60.

Frank, S. "Gamblers Anonymous," *The Saturday Evening Post,* May 26, 1962, 44–46.

Frankle, W. Gordon, Ilise Lombardo, Antonia S. New, Marianne Goodman, Peter S. Talbot, Yiyun Huang, Dah-Ren Hwang, Mark Slifstein, Susan Curry, Anissa Abi-Dargham, Marc Laruelle, and Larry J. Siever. "Brain serotonin transporter distribution in subjects with impulsive aggressivity: A positron emission study with [^{11}C] McN 5652." *American Journal of Psychiatry* 162, no. 5 (2005): 915–23.

Franko, Debra L., David J. Dorer, Pamela K. Keel, Safia Jackson, Mary Pat Manzo, and David B. Herzog. "How do eating disorders and alcohol use disorder influence each other?" *International Journal of Eating Disorders* 38, no. 3 (2000): 200–7.

Franko, Debra L., Pamela K. Keel, David J. Dorer, Mark A. Blais, Sherrie S. Delinsky, Kamryn T. Eddy, and David B. Herzog. "What predicts suicide attempts in women with eating disorders?" *Psychological Medicine* 34, no. 5 (2004): 843–53.

Frascella, Joseph, Marc N. Potenza, Lucy L. Brown, and Anna Rose Childress. "Shared brain vulnerabilities open the way for nonsubstance addictions: Carving addiction at a new joint?" *Annals of the New York Academy of Sciences* 1187 (2010): 294–315.

Gamblers Anonymous. *Sharing Recovery through Gamblers Anonymous.* Los Angeles: G. A. Publishing, 1984.

Garner, David M., Wendy Rockert, Marion P. Olmsted, Craig Johnson, and Donald V. Coscina. "Psychoeducational Principles in the Treatment of Bulimia and Anorexia Nervosa." In *Handbook of Psychotherapy for Anorexia and Bulimia,* edited by David M. Garner and Paul E. Garfinkel, 513–72. New York, NY: Guilford Press, 1985.

Gentile, Douglas. "Pathological video-game use among youth ages 8 to 18: A National Study." *Psychological Science* 20, no. 5 (2009): 594–602.

Gerstein, Dean, Sally Murphy, Marianna Toce, John Hoffman, Amanda Palmer, Robert Johnson, Cindy Larison, Lucian Chuchro, Tracy Buie, Laszlo Engelman, and Mary A. Hill. *Gambling Impact and Behavior Study: Report to the National Gambling Impact Study Commission.* Chicago: National Opinion Research Center at the University of Chicago, 1999.

Gilbert, Richard L., Nora A. Murphy, and Talisa McNally. "Addiction to the 3-dimensional internet: Estimated prevalence and relationship to real world addictions." *Addiction Research and Theory* 19, no. 4 (2011): 380–90.

Glasner-Edwards, Suzette, Larissa J. Mooney, Patricia Marinelli-Casey, Maureen Hillhouse, Alfonso Ang, Richard Rawson, and The Methamphetamine Treatment Project Corporate Authors. "Bulimia nervosa among methamphetamine dependent adults: Association with outcomes three years after treatment." *Eating Disorders* 19, no. 3 (2011): 259–69.

Godart, Nathalie T., Martine F. Flament, Y. Lecrubier, and Philippe Jeammet. "Anxiety disorders in anorexia nervosa and bulimia nervosa: Co-morbidity and chronology of appearance." *European Psychiatry* 15, no. 1 (2000): 38–45.

Goldbloom, David S., Claudio A. Naranjo, Karen E. Bremner, and Lisa K. Hicks. "Eating disorders and alcohol abuse in women." *British Journal of Addiction* 87, no. 6 (1992): 913–19.

Gonzales, Rachel, Larissa Mooney, and Richard A. Rawson. "The methamphetamine problem in the United States." *Annual Review of Public Health* 31 (2010): 385–98.

Goodman, Aviel. "Addiction: Definition and implications." *British Journal of Addiction* 85 (1990): 1403–8.

Gordon, Susan Merle, J. Aaron Johnson, Shelly F. Greenfield, Lisa Cohen, Therese Killeen, and Paul M. Roman. "Assessment and treatment of co-occurring eating disorders in publicly funded addiction treatment programs." *Psychiatric Services* 59, no. 9 (2008): 1056–59.

Grant, Jon E. *Impulse Control Disorders: A Clinician's Guide to Understanding and Treating Behavioral Addictions.* New York: W. W. Norton & Company, 2008.

Grant, Jon E. "SPECT Imaging and Treatment of Pyromania." *Journal of Clinical Psychiatry* 67, no. 6 (2006): 998.

Grant, Jon E. "The Relationship of Impulse Control Disorders to Drug and Alcohol Addiction." In *Impulse Control Disorders: A Clinician's Guide to Understanding and Treating Behavioral Addictions*, New York, NY: W.W. Norton & Company, 2008.

Grant, Jon E., Stephen Correia, and Thea Brennan-Krohn. "White matter integrity in kleptomania: A pilot study." *Psychiatry Research: Neuroimaging* 147, nos. 2–3 (2006): 233–37.

Grant, Jon E., and Suck Won Kim. "Clinical characteristics and psychiatric comorbidity of pyromania." *Journal of Clinical Psychiatry* 68 (2007): 1717–22.

Grant, Jon E., Suck Won Kim, and Brian Odlaug. "A double-blind, placebo-controlled study of the opiate antagonist, naltrexone, in the treatment of kleptomania." *Biological Psychiatry* 65, no. 7 (2009): 600–606.

Grant, Jon E., Laura Levine, Daniel Kim, and Marc N. Potenza. "Impulse control disorders in adult psychiatric inpatients." *American Journal of Psychiatry* 162, no. 11 (2005): 2184–88.

Grant, Jon E., and Brian L. Odlaug. "Clinical characteristics of trichotillomania with trichophagia." *Comprehensive Psychiatry* 49, no. 6 (2008): 579–84.

Grant, Jon E., Brian L. Odlaug, and Suck Won Kim. "N-Acetylcysteine, a glutamate modulator, in the treatment of trichotillomania." *Archives of General Psychiatry* 66, no. 7 (2009): 756–63.

Grant, Jon E., Brian L. Odlaug, and Jeffrey R. Wozniak. "Neuropsychological functioning in kleptomania." *Behavior Research and Therapy* 45, no. 7 (2007): 1663–70.

Grant Jon E., and Marc N. Potenza. "Gender-related differences in individuals seeking treatment for kleptomania." *CNS Spectrum* 13, no. 3 (2008): 235–45.

Grant, Jon E., Marc N. Potenza, Aviv Weinstein, and David A. Gorelick. "Introduction to behavioral addictions." *The American Journal of Drug and Alcohol Abuse* 36, no. 5 (2010): 233–41.

Grant, Jon E., and Marvin A. Steinberg. "Compulsive sexual behavior and pathological gambling." *Sexual Addiction & Compulsivity* 12 (2005): 235–44.

Grant, Jon E., Dan J. Stein, Douglas W. Wood, and Nancy J. Keuthen, eds., *Trichotillomania, Skin Picking & Other Body-Focused Repetitive Behaviors*, Chap. 9-12. Washington DC: American Psychiatric Publishing, Inc., 2012.

Grant, Jon E., Kyle A. Williams, and Marc N. Potenza. "Impulse control disorders in adolescent psychiatric inpatients: Co-occurring disorders and sex differences." *Journal of Clinical Psychiatry* 68 (2007): 1584–92.

Greenfield, Shelly F., Audrey J. Brooks, Susan M. Gordon, Carla A. Green, Frankie Kropp, R. Kathryn McHugh, Melissa Lincoln, Denise Hien, and Gloria M. Miele. "Substance abuse treatment entry, retention, and outcome in women: A review of the literature." *Drug and Alcohol Dependence* 86, no. 1 (2007): 1–21.

Greenfield, Shelly F., Sudie E. Back, Katie Lawson, and Kathleen T. Brady. "Substance abuse in women." *Psychiatric Clinics of North America* 33, no. 2 (2010): 339–55.

Grilo, Carlos M., Marney A. White, and Robin M. Masheb. "DSM-IV psychiatric disorder comorbidity and its correlates in binge eating disorder." *International Journal of Eating Disorders* 42, no. 3 (2009): 228–34.

Grilo, Carlos M., Rajita Sinha, and Stephanie S. O'Malley. "Eating disorders and alcohol use disorders." *Alcohol Health and Research World* 26, no. 2 (2002): 151–60.

Gritz, Ellen R., and Lori A. Crane. "Use of diet pills and amphetamines to lose weight among smoking and nonsmoking high school seniors." *Health Psychology* 10, no. 5 (1991): 330–35.

Grüesser, Sabine, M. R. Thalemann, and M. D. Griffiths. "Excessive computer game playing: Evidence for addiction and aggression?" *CyberPsychology & Behavior* 10, no. 2 (2007): 290–92.

Gupta, Rina, and Jeffrey L. Derevensky. "A treatment approach for adolescents with gambling problems." In *Gambling Problems in Youth: Theoretical and Applied Perspectives*, edited by Jeffrey Derevensky and Rina Gupta, 165–88. New York: Kluwer Academic/Plenum Publishers, 2004.

Harvard Mental Health Letter. *Pathological Gambling.* Boston: Harvard Health Publications, Harvard Medical School, Harvard University, August 2010.

Hedlund, S., M. M. Fichter, N. Quadflieg, and C. Brandl. "Expressed emotion, family environment, and parental bonding in bulimia nervosa: A 6-year investigation," *Eating and Weight Disorders* 8, no. 1 (2003): 26–35.

Herzog, David B., Debra L. Franko, David J. Dorer, Pamela K. Keel, Safia Jackson, and Mary Pat Manzo. "Drug abuse in women with eating disorders." *International Journal of Eating Disorders* 39, no. 5 (2006): 364–68.

Hodgins, David C., and Nady el-Guebaly. "Retrospective and prospective reports of precipitants to relapse in pathological gambling." *Journal of Consulting and Clinical Psychology* 72, no. 1 (2004): 72–80.

Hodgins, David C., Chrystal Mansley, and Kylie Thygesen. "Risk factors for suicide ideation and attempts among pathological gamblers." *The American Journal of Addictions* 15, no. 4 (2006): 303–10.

Holden, Constance. "Behavioral Addictions: Do they exist?" *Science* 294, no 5544 (2001): 980–82.

Holderness, Claire C., Jeanne Brooks-Gunn, and Michelle P. Warren. "Co-morbidity of eating disorders and substance abuse: Review of the literature." *International Journal of Eating Disorders* 16, no. 1 (1994): 1–34.

Hollander, Eric, Bryann Baker, Jessica Kahn, and Dan Stein. "Conceptualizing and Assessing Impulse-Control Disorders." In *Clinical Manual of Impulse-Control Disorders,* edited by Eric Hollander and Dan Stein. Washington DC: American Psychiatric Publishing, Inc., 2006.

Hollander, Eric, Heather Berlin, and Dan Stein. "Impulse-control disorders not elsewhere classified." In *The American Psychiatric Publishing Textbook of Psychiatry,* 5th ed., by Marc Galanter and Herbert D. Kleber. Washington, DC: American Psychiatric Publishing, Inc., 2008.

Hoste, Renee R. and Daniel le Grange. "Expressed emotion among white and ethnic minority families of adolescents with bulimia nervosa." *European Eating Disorders Review* 16, no. 5 (2008): 395–400.

Hrabosky, Joshua I., Robin M. Masheb, Marney A. White, and Carlos M. Grilo. "Overvaluation of shape and weight in binge eating disorder." *Journal of Consulting and Clinical Psychology* 75, no. 1 (2007): 175–80.

Hudson, James I., Eva Hiripi, Harrison G. Pope, Jr., and Ronald C. Kessler. "The prevalence and correlates of eating disorders in the National Comorbidity Survey Replication." *Biological Psychiatry* 61, no. 3 (2007): 348–58.

Hudson, James I., Harrison G. Pope Jr., Jeffrey M. Jonas, and Deborah Yurgelun-Todd. "Family history study of anorexia nervosa and bulimia." *British Journal of Psychiatry* 142 (1983): 133–38.

Hurley, Robin A., Ronald E. Fisher, and Katherine H. Taber. "Clinical and Functional Imaging in Neuropsychiatry." In *Essentials of Neuropsychiatry and Behavioral Neurosciences*. 2nd ed., edited by Stuart C. Yudofsky and Robert E. Hales, 55–94. Washington DC: American Psychiatric Publishing Inc., 2010.

Iancu, Iulian, Katherine Lowengrub, Yael Dembinsky, Moshe Kotler, and Pinhas N. Dannon. "Pathological Gambling: An update on neuropathophysiology and pharmacotherapy." *CNS Drugs* 22, no. 2 (2008): 123–38.

Illinois Department on Aging. "Action vs. escape gamblers." Illinois Department on Aging, 2005. http://www.state.il.us/aging/3hot/gambling_act-esc.htm (accessed June 11, 2012).

"Impulse-Control Disorders Not Elsewhere Classified." In *Kaplan & Sadock's Synopsis of Psychiatry: Behavioral Sciences/Clinical Psychiatry* 10th ed., by Benjamin J. Sadock and Virginia A. Sadock. Philadelphia, PA: Lippincott Williams & Wilkins, 2007.

Jacobs, Durand F. "Youth gambling in North America: Long-term trends and future prospects." In *Gambling Problems in Youth: Theoretical and Applied Perspectives*, edited by Jeffrey L. Derevensky and Rina Gupta, 1-26. New York: Kluwer Academic/Plenum Publishers, 2004.

Jeffery, Robert W., Deborah J. Hennrikus, Harry A. Lando, David M. Murray, and Jane W. Liu. "Reconciling conflicting findings regarding post-cessation weight concerns and success in smoking cessation." *Health Psychology* 19, no. 3 (2000): 242–46.

Joe, Karen A. "Ice is strong enough for a man, but made for a woman: A social cultural analysis of crystal methamphetamine use among Asian Pacific Americans." *Crime, Law and Social Change* 22, no. 3 (1995): 269–89.

Joe, Karen A. "The lives and times of Asian-Pacific American women drug users: An ethnographic study of their methamphetamine use." *Journal of Drug Issues* 26, no. 1 (1996): 199–218.

Johansson, Agneta, Jon E. Grant, Suck Won Kim, Brian L. Odlaug, and K. Gunnar Götestam. "Risk factors for problematic gambling: A critical literature review." *Journal of Gambling Studies* 25 (2009): 67–92.

Johnson, Patrick B., and Micheline S. Malow-Iroff. *Adolescents and Risk: Making Sense of Adolescent Psychology: Making Sense of Psychology*, Carol Korn-Bursztyn, Series Editor. Wetport, CT: Praeger Publishers, 2008.

Kalivas, Peter W., and Nora D. Volkow. "The neural basis of addiction: A pathology of motivation and choice." *American Journal of Psychiatry* 162, no. 8 (2005): 1403–13.

Karim, Reef, and Priya Chaudhri. "Behavioral addictions: An overview." *Journal of Psychoactive Drugs* 44, no. 1 (2012): 5–17.

Katzman, Melanie A., Art Greenberg, and Ivy D. Marcus. "Bulimia in opiate-addicted women: Developmental cousin and relapse factor." *Journal of Substance Abuse Treatment* 8, no. 3 (1991): 107–12.

Kausch, Otto. "Patterns of substance abuse among treatment-seeking pathological gamblers." *Journal of Substance Abuse Treatment* 25, no. 4 (2003): 263–70.

Kausch, Otto, Loreen Rugle, and Douglas Y. Rowland. "Lifetime histories of trauma among pathological gamblers." *The American Journal on*

Addictions 15, no. 1 (2006): 35–43.

Kaye, Walter H., Allan S. Kaplan, and Murray L. Zucker. "Treating eating-disorder patients in a managed care environment: Contemporary American issues and a Canadian response." *Psychiatric Clinics of North America* 19, no. 4 (1996): 793–810.

Kaye, Walter H., Cynthia M. Bulik, Laura Thornton, Nicole Barbarich, and Kim Masters. "Comorbidity of anxiety disorders with anorexia and bulimia nervosa." *American Journal of Psychiatry* 161 (2004): 2215–21.

Kendzor, Darla E., Lauren E. Baillie, Claire E. Adams, Diana W. Stewart, and Amy L. Copeland. "The effect of food deprivation on cigarette smoking in females." *Addictive Behavior* 33, no. 10 (2008): 1353–59.

Killen, Joel D., C. Barr Taylor, Michael J. Telch, Thomas N. Robinson, David J. Maron, and Keith E. Saylor. "Depressive symptoms and substance use among adolescent binge eaters and purgers: A defined population study." *American Journal of Public Health* 77, no. 12 (1987): 1539–41.

Kindt, John W. "The failure to regulate the gambling industry effectively: Incentives for perpetual non-compliance." *Southern Illinois University Law Journal* 27 (2002): 221–62.

Ko, Chih-Hung, Gin-Chung Liu, Sigmund Hsiao, Ju-Yu Yen, Ming-Jen Yang, Wei-Chen Lin, Cheng-Fang Yen, and Cheng-Sheng Chen. "Brain activities associated with gaming urge of online gaming addiction." *Journal of Psychiatric Research* 43, no. 7 (2009): 739–47.

Kog, Elly, and Walter Vandereycken. "Family interaction in eating disorder patients and normal controls." *International Journal of Eating Disorders* 8, no. 1 (1989): 11–23.

Koob, George F., and Michel Le Moal. "Drug addiction, dysregulation of reward, and allostasis." *Neuropsychopharmacology* 24, no. 2 (2001): 97–129.

Koob, George F., and Michel Le Moal. *Neurobiology of Addiction.* London: Elsevier, 2006.

Koran, Lorrin M., Dana Bodnik, and Pinhas N. Dannon. "Kleptomania: Clinical Aspects." In *Impulse Control Disorders*, edited by Elias Aboujaoude and Lorrin Koran. New York: Cambridge University Press, 2010.

Kormas, Georgios, Elena Critselis, Mari Janikian, Dimitrios Kafetzis, and Artemis Tsitsika. "Risk factors and psychosocial characteristics of potential problematic and problematic Internet use among adolescents: A cross-sectional study." *BioMed Central Public Health* 11, res. art. 595 (2011): 1–8. http://www.biomedcentral.com/1471-2458/11/595.

Krahn, Dean D. "The relationship between eating disorders and substance abuse." *Journal of Substance Abuse* 3, no. 2 (1991): 239–53.

Krahn, Dean D., Candace Kurth, Mark Demitrack, and Adam Drewnowski. "The relationship of dieting severity and bulimic behaviors to alcohol and other drug use in young women." *Journal of Substance Abuse* 4, no. 4 (1992): 341–53.

Kuehn, Bridget M. "Integrated care key for patients with both addiction and mental illness." *The Journal of the American Medical Association* 303, no. 19 (2010): 1905–7.

Kuss, Daria J., and Mark D. Griffiths. "Online social networking and addiction—A review of the psychological literature." *International Journal of Environmental Research and Public Health* 8 (2011): 3528–52.

Ladd, George T., and Nancy M. Petry. "Gender differences among pathological gamblers seeking treatment." *Experimental and Clinical Psychopharmacology* 10, no. 3 (2002): 302–9.

Ladouceur, Robert, and Michael B. Walker. "Cognitive approach to understanding and treating pathological gambling." In *Comprehensive*

Clinical Psychology, edited by Allen S. Bellack and Michel Hersen, 587–601, New York: Pergamon, 1998.

Ladouceur, Robert, and Stella LaChance. *Overcoming Pathological Gambling: A Therapist Guide*. New York: Oxford University Press, 2007.

Ladouceur, Robert, Caroline Sylvain, Claude Boutin, and Celine Doucet. *Understanding and Treating the Pathological Gambler*. West Sussex: John Wiley & Sons, Inc., 2003.

Lam, Lawrence T., Zi-wen Peng, Jin-cheng Mai, and Jin Jing. "Factors associated with Internet addiction among adolescents." *CyberPsychology & Behavior* 12, no. 5 (2009): 551-55.

Landau, Judith, James Garrett, and Robert Webb. "Assisting a concerned person to motivate someone experiencing cybersex into treatment: Application of invitational intervention: The ARISE model to cybersex." *Journal of Marital and Family Therapy* 34, no. 4 (2008): 498–511.

Lavik, N. J., S. E. Clausen, and W. Pedersen. "Eating behavior, drug use, psychopathology, and parental bonding in adolescents in Norway." *ActaPsychiatrica Scandinavia* 84 (1991): 387–90.

Le Grange, Daniel, Ivan Eisler, Christopher Dare, and Matthew Hodes. "Family criticism and self-starvation: A study of expressed emotion." *Journal of Family Therapy* 14 (1992): 177–92.

Lee, Shirley, and Avis Mysyk. "The medicalization of compulsive buying." *Social Science & Medicine* 58, no. 9 (2004): 1709–18.

Lee, Tayla T. C., Kristine A. Ritchey, Jonathan D. Forbey, and George A. Gaither. "Psychometrics and comparison of the compulsive sexual behavior inventory and the sexual compulsivity scale in a male college student sample." *Sexual Addiction & Compulsivity* 16, no. 2 (2009): 146–67.

Lee, Tiffany, and Angela Kent. "Sexual addiction: Screening, assessment, diagnostic criteria, and treatment options." Presentation at the Annual Conference of the American Counseling Association, Pittsburgh, PA, March 2010. Western Michigan University, 2010.

Leedes, Richard. "The three most important criteria in diagnosing sexual addictions: Obsession, obsession, and obsession." *Sexual Addiction & Compulsivity* 8 (2001): 215–26.

Lejoyeux, Michel, Nathalie Feuché, Sabrina Loi, Jacquelyn Solomon, and Jean Adès. "Study of impulsive-control disorders among alcohol-dependent patients." *Journal of Clinical Psychiatry* 60 (1999): 302–5.

Lesieur, Henry R., and Sheila B. Blume. "Pathological gambling, eating disorders, and the psychoactive substance use disorders." *Comorbidity of Addictive and Psychiatric Disorders* 12, no. 3 (1993): 89–102.

Lesieur, Henry R., and Sheila Blume. "When Lady Luck loses: Women and Compulsive Gambling." In *Feminist Perspectives on Addictions,* edited by Nan Van Den Bergh, 181–97, New York: Springer, 1991.

Lightsey, Owen Richard Jr., and C. Duncan Hulsey. "Impulsivity, coping, stress, and problem gambling among university students." *Journal of Counseling Psychology* 49, no. 2 (2002): 202–11.

Lin, Chien-Hsin, Shong-Lin Lin, and Chin-Pi Wu. "The effects of parental monitoring and leisure boredom on adolescents' internet addiction." *Adolescence* 44, no. 176 (2009): 993–1004.

Lin, Min-Pei, Huei-Chen Ko, and Jo Yung-Wei Wu. "Prevalence and psychosocial risk factors associated with Internet addiction in a nationally representative sample of college students in Taiwan." *CyberPsychology, Behavior and Social Networking* 14, no. 12 (2011): 741–46.

Linden, Robert D., Harrison G. Pope, and Jeffrey M. Jonas. "Pathological gambling and major affective disorder: Preliminary findings." *Journal of Clinical Psychiatry* 47, no. 4 (1986): 201–3.

Lingswiler, V. M., J. H. Crowther, and M. A. Stephens. "Affective and cognitive antecedents to eating episodes in bulimia and binge eating." *International Journal of Eating Disorders* 8, no. 5 (1989): 533–39.

Lipinski, Damon, James P. Whelan, and Andrew W. Meyers. "Treatment of pathological gambling using a guided self-change approach." *Clinical Case Studies* 6, no. 5 (2007): 394–411.

Marks, Isaac. "Editorial: Behavioural (non-chemical) addictions." *British Journal of Addiction* 85, no. 11 (1990): 1389–94.

Marlatt, G. Alan, and Judith R. Gordon, eds. *Relapse Prevention: Maintenance Strategies in the Treatment of Addictive Behaviors.* New York: Guilford Press, 1985.

Marrazzi, Mary Ann, and Elliot D. Luby. "An auto-addiction opioid model of chronic anorexia nervosa." *International Journal of Eating Disorders* 5, no. 2 (1986): 191–208.

Martin, Peter R., and Nancy Petry. "Are non-substance-related addictions really addictions?" *The American Journal on Addictions* 14 (2005): 1–7.

Mathes, Wendy F., Kimberly A. Brownley, Xiaofei Mo, and Cynthia M. Bulik. "The biology of binge eating." *Appetite* 52, no. 3 (2009): 545–53.

McAleavey, Kristen M., and Mary C. Fiumara. "Eating disorders: Are they addictions? A dialogue." *Journal of Social Work Practice in Addictions* 1, no. 2 (2001): 107-13.

McAllister, A. Kimberly, W. Martin Usrey, Stephen C. Noctor, and Stephen Rayport. "Fundamentals of Cellular Neurobiology." In *Essentials of Neuropsychiatry and Behavioral Neurosciences,* edited by Stuart C. Yudofsky and Robert E. Hales. Washington DC: American Psychiatric Publishing, Inc., 2010.

McCloskey, Michael S., Kurtis L. Noblett, Jerry L. Deffenbacher, Jackie K. Gollan, and Emil F. Coccaro. "Cognitive-behavioral therapy for intermittent explosive disorder: A pilot randomized clinical trial." *Journal of Consulting and Clinical Psychology* 76, no. 5 (2008): 876–86.

McCown, William George, and Linda L. Chamberlain. *Best Possible Odds: Contemporary Treatment Strategies for Gambling Disorders.* New York: John Wiley & Sons, 2000.

McDaniel, Stephen R., and Marvin Zuckerman. "The relationship of impulsive sensation seeking and gender to interest and participation in gambling activities." *Personality and Individual Differences* 35, no. 6 (2003): 1385–1400.

Merikangas, Kathleen R., Marilyn Stolar, Denise E. Stevens, Joseph Goulet, Martin A. Preisig, Brenda Fenton, Heping Zhang, Stephanie S. O'Malley, and Bruce J. Rounsaville. "Familial transmission of substance use disorders." *Archives of General Psychiatry* 55 (1998): 973–79.

Messias, Erick, Juan Castro, Anil Saini, Manzoor Usman, and Dale Peeples. "Sadness, suicide, and their association with video game and internet overuse among teens: Results from the Youth Risk Behavior Survey 2007 and 2009." *Suicide and Life-Threatening Behavior* 41, no. 3 (2011): 307–15.

Miele, Gloria M., Sarah M. Tilly, Michael First, and Allen Frances. "The definition of dependence and behavioural addictions." *British Journal of Addiction* 85 (1990): 1421–23.

Minuchin, Salvador, Bernice L. Rosman, and Lester Baker. *Psychosomatic Families: Anorexia Nervosa in Context.* Cambridge, MA: Harvard University Press, 1978.

Mitchell, James E., Melissa Burgard, Ron Faber, Ross D. Crosby, and Martina de Zwaan, "Cognitive behavioral therapy for compulsive buying disorder." *Behaviour Research and Therapy* 44, no. 12 (2006): 1859–65.

Morahan-Martin, Janet, and Phyllis Schumacher. "Incidence and correlates of pathological internet use among college students." *Computers in Human Behavior* 16, no. 1 (2000): 13–29.

Mutschler, Jochen, Mira Bühler, Martin Grosshans, Alexander Diehl, Karl Mann, and Falk Kiefer. "Disulfiram: an option for the treatment of pathological gambling?" *Alcohol and Alcoholism* 45, no. 2 (2010): 214–16.

Nabuco de Abreu, Christiano, and Dora Sampaio Goes. "Psychotherapy for internet addiction." In *Internet Addiction: A Handbook and Guide to Evaluation and Treatment* edited by Kimberly S. Young and Christiano Nabuco de Abreu. Hoboken, NJ: John Wiley & Sons, Inc., 2011.

National Gambling Impact Study Commission (NGISC). *Final Report.* Washington DC: Government Printing Office, 1999.

National Research Council (NRC), *Pathological Gambling: A Critical Review.* Washington DC: National Academy Press, 1999.

Neal, Alice, Suzanne Abraham, and Janice Russell. "'Ice' use and eating disorders: A report of three cases." *International Journal of Eating Disorders* 42, no. 2 (2009): 188–91.

Nestler, Eric J. and David W. Self. "Neuropsychiatric Aspects of Ethanol and Other Chemical Dependencies." In *Essentials of Neuropsychiatry and Behavioral Neurosciences*, edited by Stuart C. Yudofsky and Robert E. Hales. Washington DC: American Psychiatric Publishing, Inc., 2010.

Nower, Lia. "Pathological gamblers in the workplace: A primer for employers." *Employee Assistance Quarterly* 18, no. 4 (2003): 55–72.

Nower, Lia, and Alex Blaszczynski. "A pathways approach to treating youth gamblers." In *Gambling Problems in Youth: Theoretical and Applied Perspectives*, edited by Jeffrey L. Derevensky and Rina Gupta, 189–209. New York: Kluwer Academic/Plenum Publishers, 2004.

Nower, Lia, and Alex Blaszczynski. "Recovery in pathological gambling: An imprecise concept." *Substance Use and Misuse* 43, no. 12–13 (2008): 1844–64.

Odlaug, Brian L., and Jon E. Grant. "Impulse-control disorders in a college sample: Results from the self-administered Minnesota Impulse Disorders Interview (MIDI)." *Primary Care Companion Journal of Clinical Psychiatry* 12, no. 2 (2010): e1–e5.

Oei, Tian P. S., and Leon M. Gordon. "Psychosocial factors related to gambling abstinence and relapse in members of Gamblers Anonymous." *Journal of Gambling Studies* 24, no. 1 (2008): 91–105.

Okon, Deborah, Anita L. Greene and Jane E. Smith. "Family interactions predict intra-individual symptom variation for adolescents with bulimia." *International Journal of Eating Disorders* 34, no. 4 (2003): 450–57.

Olsen, Christopher M. "Natural rewards, neuroplasticity, and non-drug addictions." *Neuropharmacology* 61, no. 7 (2011): 1109–22.

Park, Soo Kyung, Jae Yop Kim, and Choon Bum Cho. "Prevalence of Internet addiction and correlations with family factors among South Korean adolescents." *Adolescence* 43, no. 172 (2009): 895–909.

Parker, Jan, and Diana Guest. "Individual sexual addiction treatment: A developmental perspective." *Sexual Addiction & Compulsivity* 10, no. 1 (2003): 13–23.

Parkes, Sarah P., Elizabeth M. Saewyc, David N. Cox, and Laura J. MacKay. "Relationship between body image and stimulant use among Canadian adolescents." *Journal of Adolescent Health* 43, no. 6 (2008): 616–18.

Petry, Nancy M. "Commentary on Van Rooij et al. (2011): 'Gaming addiction'–a psychiatric disorder or not?" *Addiction* 106, no. 1 (2011): 213–14.

Petry, Nancy M. *Pathological Gambling: Etiology, Comorbidity, and Treatment.* Washington DC: American Psychological Association, 2005.

Petry, Nancy M., Mark D. Litt, Ronald Kadden, and David M. Ledgerwood. "Do coping skills mediate the relationship between cognitive-behavioral therapy and reductions in gambling in pathological gamblers?" *Addiction* 102, no. 8 (2007): 1280–91.

Peveler, Robert, and Christopher Fairburn. "Eating disorders in women who abuse alcohol." *British Journal of Addiction* 85, no. 12 (1990): 1633–38.

Phillips, Denise. "Gambling: The hidden addiction: Cases of this psychiatric disorder are on the rise as more Americans fall under the spell of 'Lady Luck' (Addictions)," *Behavioral Health Management*, September 2005, 32–37.

Pies, Ronald. "Should DSM-V designate "internet addiction" a mental disorder?" *Psychiatry* 6, no. 2 (2009): 31–37.

Pike, K. M., A Hilbert, Denise E. Wilfley, C. G. Fairburn, F. A. Dohm, B. T. Walsh, and R. H. Striegel-Moore. "Toward an understanding of risk factors for anorexia nervosa: A case-controlled study." *Psychological Medicine* 38, no. 10 (2008): 1443–53.

Pilkonis, Paul A., Hilary Feldman, and Jonathan Himmelhoch. "Social anxiety and substance abuse in affective disorders." *Comprehensive Psychiatry* 22, no. 5 (1981): 451–57.

Pillitteri, Janine L., Saul Shiffman, Jeffrey M. Rohay, Andrea M. Harkins, Steven L. Burton, and Thomas A. Wadden. "Use of dietary supplements for weight loss in the United States: Results of a national survey." *Obesity* 16, no. 4 (2008): 790–96.

Piran, Niva, and Shannon R. Robinson. "The association between disordered eating and substance use and abuse in women: A community-based investigation." *Women and Health* 44, no. 1 (2006): 1–20.

Pisetsky, Emily M., Y. May Chao, Lisa C. Dierker, Alexis M. May, and Ruth H. Striegel-Moore. "Disordered eating and substance use in high school students: Results from the youth risk behavior surveillance system." *International Journal of Eating Disorders* 41, no. 5 (2008): 464–70.

Plant, Martin, and Moira Plant. "Sex addiction: A comparison with dependence on psychoactive drugs." *Journal of Substance Use* 8, no. 4 (2003): 260–66.

Potenza, Marc N. "The neurobiology of pathological gambling and drug addiction: An overview and new findings." *Philosophical Transactions of the Royal Society B (Biological Sciences)* 363 (2008): 3181–89.

Potenza, Marc N., Lorrin M. Koran, and Stefano Pallanti. "The relationship between impulse-control disorders and obsessive-compulsive disorder: A current understanding and future research directions." *Psychiatry Research* 170, no. 1 (2009): 22–31.

Power, Cynthia. "Food and sex addiction: Helping the clinician recognize and treat the interaction." *Sexual Addiction & Compulsivity* 12 (2005): 219–34.

Redgrave, Graham W., Janelle W. Coughlin, Leslie J. Heinberg, and Angela S. Guarda. "First- degree relative history of alcoholism in eating disorder inpatients: Relationship to eating and substance use pathology." *Eating Behaviors* 8, no. 1 (2007): 15–22.

Reece, Michael, and Brian Dodge. "Exploring indicators of sexual compulsivity among men who cruise for sex on campus." *Sexual Addiction & Compulsivity* 11 (2004): 87–113.

Root, Tammy L., Andréa P. Pinheiro, Laura Thornton, Michael Strober, Fernando Fernandez-Aranda, Harry Brandt, Steve Crawford, et al. "Substance use disorders in women with anorexia nervosa." *International Journal of Eating Disorders* 43, no. 1 (2010): 14–21.

Ruschmann, Paul. *Legalized Gambling*. New York, NY: Chelsea House Publishers, 2009.

Sachs, Kenneth S. "Psychotherapy and Alcoholics Anonymous: A guide for therapists." *Alcoholism Treatment Quarterly* 27, no. 2 (2009): 199–212.

Sang-Hun, Choe. "South Korea Expands Aid for Internet Addiction." *New York Times*, May 28, 2010. http://www.nytimes.com/2010/05/29/world/asia/29game.html (accessed March 29, 2012).

Schreiber, Liana, Brian L. Odlaug, and Jon E. Grant. "Impulse control disorders: Updated review of clinical characteristics and pharmacological management." *Frontiers in Psychiatry* 2, art. 1 (2011): 1–11.

Schwer, R. Keith, William N. Thompson, and Daryl Nakamuro. "Beyond the limits of recreation: Social costs of gambling in Southern Nevada." Paper presented at the annual meeting of the Far West and American Popular Culture Association, Las Vegas, NV, February 1, 2003.

Shaffer, Howard J., and Matthew N. Hall. "Updating and refining prevalence estimates of disordered gambling behavior in the United States and Canada." *Canadian Journal of Public Health* 92, no. 3 (2001): 168–72.

Shaffer, Howard J., and David A. Korn. "Gambling and related mental disorders: A public health analysis." *Annual Review of Public Health* 23 (2002): 171–212.

Shaffer, Howard J., Debi A. LaPlante, Richard A. LaBrie, Rachel C. Kidman, Anthony N. Donato, and Michael V. Stanton. "Toward a syndrome model of addiction: Multiple expressions, common etiology." *Harvard Review of Psychiatry* 12 (2004): 367–74.

Shapira, Nathan A., Mary C. Lessig, Toby D. Goldsmith, Steven T. Szabo, Martin Lazoritz, Mark S. Gold, and Dan J. Stein. "Problematic internet use: Proposed classification and diagnostic criteria." *Depression and Anxiety* 17, no. 4 (2003): 207–16.

Sharpe, Louise. "A reformulated cognitive-behavioral model of problem gambling: A biopsychosocial perspective." *Clinical Psychology Review* 22, no. 1 (2002): 1–25.

Shaw, Martha, and Donald W. Black. "Internet addiction: Definition, assessment, epidemiology and clinical management." *CNS Drugs* 22, no. 5 (2008): 353–65.

Sherman, Susan G., Danielle German, Bangorn Sirirojn, Nick Thompson, Apinun Aramrattana, and David D. Celentano. "Initiation of methamphetamine use among young Thai drug users: A qualitative study." *Journal of Adolescent Health* 42, no. 1 (2008): 36–42.

Siever, Larry J. "Neurobiology of aggression and violence." *American Journal of Psychiatry* 165, no. 4 (2008): 429–42.

Slutske, Wendy S. "Natural recovery and treatment-seeking in pathological gambling: Results of two U.S. national surveys." *American Journal of Psychiatry* 163, no. 2 (2006): 297–302.

Soh, Nerissa L., Stephen W. Touyz, and Lois J. Surgenor. "Eating and body image disturbances across cultures: A review." *European Eating Disorders Review* 14, no. 1 (2006): 54–65.

Spooner, Lauren C., and William J. Lyddon. "Sandtray therapy for inpatient sexual addiction treatment: An application of constructivist change principles." *Journal of Constructivist Psychology* 20, no. 1 (2007): 53–85.

Stewart, Sherry H., Catrina G. Brown, Kristina Devoulyte, Jennifer Theakston, and Sarah E. Larsen. "Why do women with alcohol problems binge eat? Exploring connections between binge eating and heavy drinking in women receiving treatment for alcohol problems." *Journal of Health Psychology* 11, no. 3 (2006): 409–25.

Stewart, Sherry H., Maria Angelopoulos, Jan M. Baker, and Fred J. Boland "Relations between dietary restraint and patterns of alcohol use in young adult women." *Psychology of Addictive Behaviors* 14, no. 1 (2000): 77–82.

Stock, Suzanne L., Eudice Goldberg, Shannon Corbett, and Debra K. Katzmann. "Substance use in female adolescents with eating disorders." *Journal of Adolescent Health* 31, no. 2 (2002): 176–82.

Striegel-Moore, Ruth H., and Debra L. Franko. "Should binge eating disorder be included in the DSM-V? A critical review of the state of the evidence." *Annual Review of Clinical Psychology* 4, (2008): 305–24.

Striegel-Moore, Ruth H., and Edward S. Huydic. "Problem drinking and symptoms of disordered eating in female high school students." *International Journal of Eating Disorders* 14, no. 4 (1993): 417–25.

Streifel, Cathy, and Heather Servanty-Seib. "Alcoholics Anonymous: Novel applications of two theories." *Alcoholism Treatment Quarterly* 24, no. 3 (2006): 71–91.

Striegel-Moore, Ruth H., Lisa R. Silberstein, and Judith Rodin. "The social self in bulimia nervosa: Public self-consciousness, social anxiety, and perceived fraudulence." *Journal of Abnormal Psychology* 102, no. 2 (1993): 297–303.

Strober, Michael. "The significance of bulimia in juvenile anorexia nervosa: An exploration of possible etiologic factors." *International Journal of Eating Disorders* 1, no. 1 (1981): 28–43.

Strober, Michael, Roberta Freeman, Stacy Bower, and Joanne Kigali. "Binge eating in anorexia nervosa predicts later onset of substance use disorder: A ten-year prospective, longitudinal follow-up of 95 adolescents." *Journal of Youth and Adolescence* 25, no. 4 (1996): 519–32.

Substance Abuse and Mental Health Services Administration, Office of Applied Studies. "Results from the 2007 National Survey on Drug Use and Health: National Findings" (NSDUH Series H-34, DHHS Publication No. SMA 08-4343). Rockville, MD. US Department of Health and Human Services, http: //www. samhsa.gov/data/nsduh/2k7nsduh 2k7results.pdf (accessed June 11, 2012).

Suurvali, Helen, David C. Hodgins, and John A. Cunningham. "Motivators for resolving or seeking help for gambling problems: A review of the empirical literature," *Journal of Gambling Studies* 26 (2010): 1–33.

Sysko, Robyn, and Tom Hildebrandt. "Cognitive-behavioural therapy for individuals with bulimia nervosa and a co-occurring substance use disorder." *European Eating Disorders Review* 17, no. 2 (2009): 89–100.

Szmukler, George I., and Digby Tantam. "Anorexia nervosa: Starvation dependence." *British Journal of Psychology* 57, no. 4 (1984): 303–10.

Szmukler, George I., R. Berkowitz, Ivan Eisler, J. Leff, and Christopher Dare. "Expressed emotion in individual and family settings: A comparative study." *British Journal of Psychiatry* 151 (1987): 174–78.

Talih, Farid Ramzi. "Kleptomania and potential exacerbating factors: A review and case report." *Innovations in Clinical Neuroscience* 8, no. 10 (2011): 35–39.

The National Center on Addiction and Substance Abuse (CASA) at Columbia University. (2003). *Food for thought: Substance abuse and eating disorders.* Retrieved from http://www.casacolumbia.org/templates/Publications_ Reports.aspx

Thornton, Christopher, and Janice Russell. "Obsessive-compulsive comorbidity in the dieting disorders." *International Journal of Eating Disorders* 21, no. 1 (1997): 83–87.

Toneatto, Tony, and Robert Ladoceur. "The treatment of pathological gambling: A critical review of the literature." *Psychology of Addictive Behaviors* 17 (2003): 284–92.

Trainor, Kathleen. "Treating Trichotillomania in Children and Adolescents: CBT Versus Medication." *American Journal of Psychiatry* 164, no. 10 (2007): 1610–11.

Tsai, Hsing Fang, Chu Hui Cheng, Tzung Lieh Yeh, Chi-Chen Shih, Kao Ching Chen, Yi Ching Yang, and Yen Kuang Yang. "The risk factors of Internet addiction—A survey of university freshmen." *Psychiatry Research* 167, no. 3 (2009): 294–99.

Turner, Nigel E., Umesh Jain, Warren Spence, and Masood Zangeneh. "Pathways to pathological gambling: Component analysis of variables related to pathological gambling." *International Gambling Studies* 8, no. 3 (2008): 281–98.

Valenti, Suaye Anna Maria. "Use of object relations and self-psychology as treatment for sex addiction with a female borderline patient." *Sexual Addiction & Compulsivity* 9, no. 4 (2002): 249–62.

Van Rooij, Antonius J., Tim M. Schoenmakers, Regina J. J. M. van de Eijnden, and Dick van de Mheen. "Compulsive internet use: The role of online gaming and other Internet applications." *Journal of Adolescent Health* 47, no. 1 (2010): 51–57.

Virkkunen, Matti, Monika Eggert, Robert Rawlings, and Markku Linnoila. "A prospective follow-up study of alcoholic violent offenders and fire setters." *Archives of General Psychiatry* 53 (1996): 523–29.

Volberg, Rachel A. "The prevalence and demographics of pathological gamblers: Implications for public health." *American Journal of Public Health* 84, no. 2 (1994): 217–41.

Volkow, Nora D., Gene-Jack Wang, and Ruben D. Baler. "Reward, dopamine and the control of food intake: Implications for obesity." *Trends in Cognitive Sciences* 15, no. 1 (2011): 37–46.

Volkow, Nora D., Joanna S. Fowler, and Gene-Jack Wang. "The addicted human brain viewed in the light of imaging studies: Brain circuits and treatment strategies." *Neuropharmacology* 47, supp. 1 (2004): 3–13.

Von Mayrhauser, Christina, Mary-Lynn Brecht, and M. Douglas Anglin. "Use ecology and drug use motivations of methamphetamine users admitted to substance abuse treatment facilities in Los Angeles: An emerging profile." *Journal of Addictive Diseases* 21, no. 1 (2001): 45–60.

Walfish, Steven, David E. Stenmark, Denise Sarco, J. Steven Shealy, and Anton M. Krone. "Incidence of bulimia in substance misusing women in residential treatment." *The International Journal of the Addictions* 27, no. 4 (1992): 425–33.

Waller, Glenn and Rachel Calam. "Parenting and family factors in eating problems." In *Understanding Eating Disorders: Anorexia Nervosa, Bulimia Nervosa, and Obesity*, by LeeAnn Alexander-Mott and D. Barry Lumsden, eds., 61–76. Washington, DC: Taylor & Francis, 1994.

Walsh, B. Timothy, Steven P. Roose, Alexander H. Glassman, Madeline Gladis, and Carla Sadik. "Bulimia and depression." *Psychosomatic Medicine* 47, no. 2 (1985): 123–31.

Walther, Michael R., Benjamin T. P. Tucker, and Douglas W. Woods. "Trichotillomania: Clinical Aspects." In *Impulse Control Disorders*, edited by Elias Aboujaoude, and Lorrin M. Koran. New York: Cambridge University Press, 2010.

Wang, Hui, Xiaolan Zhou, Ciyong Lu, Jie Wu, Xueqing Deng, and Lingyao Hong. "Problematic Internet use in high school students in Guangdong Province, China." *PLoS ONE* 6, no. 5 (2011): e19660.

Welch, Sarah L., Christopher G. Fairburn. "Impulsivity or comorbidity in bulimia nervosa: A controlled study of deliberate self-harm and alcohol and drug misuse in a community sample." *British Journal of Psychiatry* 169, no. 4 (1996): 451–58.

Widyanto, Laura, and Mary McMurran. "The psychometric properties of the internet addiction test." *CyberPsychology & Behavior* 7, no. 4 (2004): 443–50.

Wilson, G. Terence. "Eating disorders and addiction." *Drugs & Society* 15, no. 1 (2000): 87–101.

Wilson, G. Terence. "Eating disorders, obesity, and addiction." *European Eating Disorders Review* 18, no. 5 (2010): 341–51.

Wilson, Marie. "Creativity and shame reduction in sex addiction treatment." *Sexual Addiction & Compulsivity* 7 (2000): 229–48.

Wise, Roy A. "Action of drugs of abuse on brain reward systems." *Pharmacology Biochemistry and Behavior* 13, supp. 1 (1980): 213–23.

Wise, Roy A. "Brain reward circuitry: Insights from unsensed incentives." *Neuron* 36 (2002): 229–40.

Wiseman, Claire V., Suzanne R. Sunday, Patricia Halligan, Suzanne Korn, Christine Brown, and Katherine A. Halmi. "Substance dependence and eating disorders: Impact of sequence on comorbidity." *Comprehensive Psychiatry* 40, no. 5 (1999): 332–36.

Wolfe, Wendy L., and Stephen A. Maisto. "The relationship between eating disorders and substance use: Moving beyond co-prevalence research." *Clinical Psychology Review* 20, no. 5 (2000): 617–31.

Wonderlich, Stephen. "Relationship of family and personality factors in bulimia." In *The Etiology of Bulimia Nervosa: The Individual and Family Context* by Janis H. Crowther, Daniel L. Tennenbaum, Steven E. Hobfoll, and Mary Ann Parris Stephens, eds., 103–126. Washington, DC: Hemisphere Publishing, 1992.

Xinaris, Skevoulla, and Frederick J. Boland. "Disordered eating in relation to tobacco use, alcohol consumption, self-control, and sex-role ideology." *International Journal of Eating Disorders* 9, no. 4 (1990): 425–43.

Yellowlees, Peter M., and Shayna Marks. "Problematic Internet use or Internet addiction?" *Computers in Human Behavior* 23, no. 3 (2007): 1447–53.

Yen, Cheng-Fang, Chih-Hung Ko, Ju-Yu Yen, Yu-Ping Chang, Chung-Ping Cheng. "Multi- dimensional discriminative factors for Internet addiction among adolescents regarding gender and age." *Psychiatry and Clinical Neurosciences* 63 (2009): 357–64.

Yen, Ju-Yu, Cheng-Fang Yen, Cheng-Chung Chen, Sue-Huei Chen, and Chih-Hung Ko. "Family factors of Internet addiction and substance use experience in Taiwanese adolescents." *CyberPsychology & Behavior* 10, no. 3 (2007): 323–29.

Yen, Ju-Yu, Chih-Hung Ko, Chen-Fang Yen, Sue-Huei Chen, Wei-Lun Chung, and Cheng-Chung Chen. "Psychiatric symptoms in adolescents with Internet addiction: Comparison with substance use." *Psychiatry and Clinical Neurosciences* 62, no. 1 (2008): 9–16.

Young, Kimberly S. "CBT-IA: The first treatment model for Internet addiction." *Journal of Cognitive Psychotherapy: An International Quarterly* 25, no. 4 (2011): 304–12.

Young, Kimberly S. "Internet sex addiction: Risk factors, stages of development, and treatment." *American Behavioral Scientist* 52, no. 1 (2008): 21–37.

Zhang, Xm-Qian, Yue-Qin Huang, Xiao-Min Luo, and Zhao-Rui Liu. "A cross-sectional study of Internet addiction disorder in high school students in Beijing." *Chinese Mental Health Journal* 23, no. 10 (2009): 748–51.

Zhong, Xin, Si Zu, Sha Sha, Ran Tao, Chongsi Zhao, Fengchi Yang, Mei Li, and Peng Sha. "The effect of a family-based intervention model on internet-addicted Chinese adolescents." *Social Behavior and Personality* 39, no. 8 (2011): 1021–34.

Zhou, Shi-jie, Zhi-hong Tang, Yang Peng. "Internet-related behavior characteristics of adolescents with Internet addiction." *Chinese Journal of Clinical Psychology* 17, no. 2 (2009): 151–153.